ROAD TO WELLNESS

Roadmap for a Lifestyle of Health

Road to Wellness packs much of Debra Raybern's clinical experience and Laura Hopkins' practical insights into a guide every family can take to truly live the abundantly healthy and vibrant life they desire. The mentor and student have collaborated on this project from their unique perspectives, preparing the reader for the possible highs and lows and the ultimate rewards of this wellness journey. It is not meant to be all-inclusive, as each person's journey is his or her own. Instead, it is the starting point for a road *well*-traveled!

Debra Raybern
Laura Hopkins

ISBN: 978-0-9816954-4-0
Printed in the United States of America
First Printing.

Growing Healthy Homes LLC
P.O. Box 3154
Bartlesville, OK 74006

To obtain additional copies of this book, please visit
www.GrowingHealthyHomes.com.

Disclaimer:
The information in this manual is for educational purposes and is not intended to diagnose, treat, or prescribe for any disease. This is a compilation of the authors' beliefs based on both independent research and professional and personal experiences. The content of this book does not necessarily reflect the views of Young Living Essential Oils, LC, Lehi, UT, (YL) and is produced by Independent Distributors. The authors, publishers, and YL bear no responsibility for the misuse of any information in this manual or the misuse of products. The choice to use or not use any of this information is the sole responsibility of the reader. The authors only endorse the use of Young Living Essential Oils because of the quality and purity of the products through the Seed to Seal® Process.

About Young Living

The authors endorse the use of Young Living Essential Oils and oil-infused products because of personal and clinical experience. This book was written with current members of Young Living in mind.

However, if you are not a member of Young Living, you should contact the person who introduced you to the oils or oil-infused products, or who gave you this book. That person should have a Young Living member number you can use to create a wholesale membership. If you do not have a Young Living contact, you can call the company, and they will recommend a leader in your region. You may also use the author's information at the back of this manual.

Young Living wholesale members receive 24% off the retail price and are eligible for the optional monthly purchasing program – Essential Rewards (ER). Debra and Laura have participated in ER for decades and enjoy the benefits of reduced shipping costs, special collections and gifts only available for ER members, and the ability to redeem ER points for products. You may enroll for ER as soon as you become a member to enjoy the benefits right away and have the products you need for the *Road to Wellness* at the best price!

We dedicate *Road to Wellness* to all those who desire to live life to the fullest! To families everywhere who have tried and failed to find a system that puts them in the driver's seat of their own wellness, we are rooting for your success! To our families who have given us time to write, have been our best "test" subjects, and became recipients of greater wellness along the way, we love and are forever grateful for you.

Debra Raybern & Laura Hopkins

Why a *Road to Wellness*?

If you don't know where you're going, any road will take you there. However, if you have a specific destination in mind, you need a specific plan and directions to get you there. Would you want to know about road closures, tolls, and possible traffic jams? We have the technology today to lead us just about anywhere in the world.

Do you have a plan to move forward in health, traversing unknown terrain and gaining knowledge to make your own personalized roadmap?

> Maybe you are already on this path and want to be more intentional.
> Maybe you know you need to begin the journey, but you don't know where to start.
> Maybe someone gave you this because they want you to join them on the journey.

Whatever your reason for opening and reading this first page, we challenge you to take action. If you're too busy, too tired, or too apathetic, you are not alone. This is your "before" snapshot, and it will make a phenomenal backstory someday. That's something your spouse, kids, siblings, and other loved ones will proudly share about you as they tell others of your healthy transformation.

We cannot just spend our days waiting to get well without taking action. In order to live and end life at the destination of health, we must make small choices daily that lead us down the Road of Wellness. It doesn't always go so smoothly, but it doesn't go at all without a plan. This manual was designed to give you strategic steps to incorporate over time that will create intentionality in your life. You simply have to use it.

Throughout Road to Wellness, you will see encouragement and additional personal details about our individual journeys. Every person has unique and relevant experiences that are his or her own; embrace the challenges and celebrate the victories along the way.

We purposefully titled this manual *Road to Wellness: Roadmap for a Lifestyle of Health* as a companion to our previous collaboration, *Road to Royal: Roadmap to Success*, for leaders pursuing abundance with Young Living Essential Oils. Like that road, we also travel this road *well*-traveled WITH you, sharing our insights from this excellent, challenging adventure. What do you gain by pursing wealth at the expense of your health? Most likely, you will spend the end of your life and all of your wealth pursuing health.

Will you determine with us that we will choose health, leaving a legacy of wellness, purpose, and abundance? You will find that your health is the greatest wealth you can attain; it may be the most profound and significant legacy you leave for future generations to inherit. Immerse yourself in your own and your family's wellness. A few changes today can make a huge impact in a lifetime of wellness. Not everything will change overnight, but if you give yourself time, things will begin to change for the better. ENJOY THE JOURNEY!

Debra Raybern & Laura Hopkins

Throughout this book, which is for everyone regardless of personal faith, we will often mention God and reference scriptures from the Bible. So, if you are unfamiliar with this, please understand that our faith flows from an exuberant love for God and the truth that He desires a relationship with each of us.

It is our prayer that you understand our perspective of health by first understanding our foundational beliefs about healing and wholeness.

We believe God created the earth and everything in it and that humans were created in the image of God to know Him intimately. We believe the victorious and redemptive work of Christ on the cross provides freedom from the power of the enemy–sin, lies, sickness, and torment. We believe that we were restored to fellowship with God through repenting, believing, and receiving Jesus as our Lord and Savior, and that this salvation is available to everyone.

Everyone sins; it's part of being a human. Because sin separates us from God, He made a way for us to be rejoined to him. We must acknowledge that our sin has separated us, ask for forgiveness, and believe that He made a way to rejoin Him.

In Romans 10:9-10 says, "If you confess with your mouth, 'Jesus is Lord,' and believe in your heart that God raised Him from the dead, you will be saved. For it is with your heart that you believe and are justified, and it is with your mouth that you confess and are saved."

To say you are justified means that you are acquitted of your sins and declared to be in right standing with God. *That's awesome!* It doesn't mean you will be perfect, but that you know that God loves you unconditionally and offers forgiveness. It also means that you can allow the Holy Spirit and the Word of God to transform you by renewing your mind. (Romans 12:2) Accepting Jesus is not a promise of an easy life, but a promise that He won't leave us or forsake us. Think of it as a caterpillar transforming into a butterfly! *Why would you go back to crawling when you know how to fly?*

Please let us know if you have accepted Jesus as Lord and joined our family! The most important thing for you to do next is to read the Bible and learn to hear God's voice daily. You also need to find people in your community who study the Bible, can walk with you, and encourage you in this journey. We are not just living for the promise of heaven someday, but to share the love of Jesus here on earth and walk in His ways now!

We believe freedom in body, mind, and spirit is His plan for you!

"If the Son sets you free, you are free indeed!"

John 8:36

Always consult a medical professional before going on a cleanse or going off any medications.

Our bodies are not deficient in medications, but due to a not-so-healthy past or unforeseen issue, symptoms arise that are addressed through medication. If you are currently taking medications, cleansing and nourishing your body may alter the working of the medication. In fact, you may notice less need for it.

At no time do the authors recommend you stop taking your prescribed medicines, but as your body begins to rejuvenate and restore itself, your dependence on them may be reduced or eliminated altogether. It is best to consult your doctor and tell him or her that you are taking steps to reduce the amount of medication you consume and to eventually eliminate the need for this medicine altogether.

Because some medications carry unwanted side effects if stopped suddenly, please consult your healthcare provider before making radical changes. Ask him or her to work *with* you to require less or even no medication and ask if he or she is willing to monitor you in this process for the next 3 to 6 months or more.

Do the authors believe that there is a time and place for modern medicine? Of course. We also believe that each of us should take a look at the state of our health, the health trends of our nation and generation, and challenge the status quo. Ask yourself …

> Should I rely on long-term usage of pharmaceuticals when proper nutrition, cleansing, and lifestyle changes can bring me freedom from medications?

> If the road that brought me to an unhealthy stage of needing medication is a literal dead end, wouldn't it be wise to reverse direction and find a healthier road to travel?

Our bodies are "fearfully and wonderfully made," and they were not created to rely on modern medicines; however, after years of using medicine regularly and experiencing toxic overloads of all varieties, your current state of health should be evaluated.

We believe that you can be an overcomer by cleansing and nourishing the whole body, mind, emotions, and spirit! Keep in mind that you didn't get to where you are overnight, nor should you expect one cleanse or a diet change to fix everything in one weekend. The healthy path is a complete lifestyle change that you can choose to journey for the rest of your life. Celebrate the milestones of getting back in the right direction and staying on track. You are worth it, and those who love you will agree!

How to Use *Road to Wellness*

1. **Passively**
   • Read the insights and suggestions to gain head knowledge, but do not make a commitment to do it. This approach will yield moderate insight. If not put into practice, this content will not change anything. You're still on a dead end road going in the wrong direction.

2. **Actively** – for the person who is ready for CHANGE!
   • Fill in the blanks and charts, and take copious notes.
   • Find friends who will keep you accountable to your plan.
   • Complete "MY PLAN" at the end of each step based on your answers on the previous pages.
   • Record your accomplishments!
   • Celebrate your accomplishments with your friends!
   • Gift a roadmap to those friends and be their accountability partner.
   • See how many loved ones you can inspire with your transformation.
   • Live a longer, healthier life to enjoy with your loved ones!

CHOOSE #2!!!

First, take inventory of yourself and your environment.
   • Rid the home of the chemicals that are harmful.
   • Next, move on to the pantry and refrigerator.
   • Then, identify and release toxic emotions.
   • Cleanse and nourish your body.
   • Lastly, add daily supplements and oils to your clean and stable foundation.

You'll notice right away that we don't start with cleansing the body or a specific organ. Why? Because you must first change your environment – namely removing the chemically-laden products you've been passively ingesting through the air you breathe as well as what you put on and in your body.

Progressing through these stages will give you the necessary framework and wisdom to keep harmful products from reentering your environment and you. Even during the first steps of cleansing your house, you may begin to see health improvements. When you incorporate a good diet, begin cleansing your insides, and add select supplements, you'll have a plan to maintain wellness.

Road to Wellness is a starting point for your journey and is not intended to be all inclusive on all topics. As you continue down this path, you will independently learn more in your environment and the foods you eat that pose a danger to your wellness, but because you started with intentional steps with this manual, you will be well informed to make long lasting, effective changes. Additional blank charts are available in the Resource Section or http://growinghealthyhomes.com/bookextras.

Seven Steps for the Road *Well* Traveled

STEP ONE
Before You Journey

STEP ONE
Before You Journey

If you don't know where you're going, any road will take you there. However, if you have a specific destination in mind, you want to travel the best roads to ensure you will arrive safely by the time you want to be there.

You must make the decision to be well.

Copy this sentence in the space below and say it out loud:

"I desire to be well and thrive in life."

_____

Now, you need to take some measurements and maybe make an appointment with a healthcare provider to get an accurate picture of your current wellness. Getting blood work done is a smart first step to determine your baseline health.

Contact your local physician or insurance agency (life insurance requires a physical exam) to get a full laboratory analysis. If you prefer to get your results without seeing a medical professional for any reason, there are several places you can still get routine blood tests, often called wellness screenings:

www.lifelinescreening.com   www.healthcheckusa.com   www.anylabtest.com

Many popular pharmacy chains and neighborhood drugstores often provide these screenings as well.

Be sure to ask for the traditional CBC (Complete Blood Chemistry), and make sure it includes a complete thyroid panel (T3, T4, T7 and TSH), not just TSH.

In addition to getting your blood work done, getting a full physical may help you assess your physical strengths. Either have your physician take the following measurements, or you can follow the directions to do so at home.

Height: _____

Weight: _____

Body Mass Index (BMI): _____

BMI determinations:
    Underweight = <18.5
    Normal weight = 18.5–24.9
    Overweight = 25–29.9
    Obesity = BMI of 30 or greater

Pulse: _____

Find your pulse on the side of the neck, the inside of the elbow, or at the wrist. For most people, it is easiest to take the pulse at the wrist. If you use the lower neck, be sure not to press too hard, and never press on the pulses on both sides of the lower neck at the same time to prevent blocking blood flow to the brain. When taking your pulse:

 • Use the first and second fingertips to press firmly yet gently on the arteries until you feel a pulse.
 • Count your pulse for 15 seconds and then multiply by four to calculate beats per minute.
 • Concentrate on the beat of the pulse rather than watching the clock

Blood pressure: _____

Use an at home digital blood pressure wrist cuff or go to a local pharmacy/grocery store and have it taken by a free machine.

Blood Pressure Category	Systolic mm Hg (upper #)		Diastolic mm Hg (upper #)
Normal	Less than 120	and	Less than 80
Prehypertension	120-139	or	80-89
High Blood Pressure (Hypertension) Stage 1	140-159	or	90-99
High Blood Pressure (Hypertension) Stage 2	160 or higher	or	100 or higher
Hypertensive Crisis Emergency care needed	Higher than 180	or	Higher than 110

Basal body temperature:_____

Anything below 97.8 is an indicator your thyroid may be low, often due to lack of iodine.

pH: _____

The ideal pH for human blood is between 7.4 and 7.6 – slightly more alkaline than acidic. You can purchase litmus-paper strips online or at some pharmacies and test your pH. When blood loses alkalinity and becomes more acidic, it creates a challenging environment for healing because an acidic environment allows unfriendly bacteria and fungi to thrive. You can achieve a balanced pH through changes in the diet, increased water intake, avoiding antibiotics, and taking control of emotions, all of which will be addressed in *Road to Wellness*.

Understanding Your Results
It's important to note here that laboratory test results reported as numbers are not meaningful by themselves. Their meaning comes from comparison to reference values. Reference values are the values expected for a healthy person. They are sometimes called "normal" values.

https://labtestsonline.org/understanding/features/ref-ranges

A reference range is a set of values that includes upper and lower limits of a lab test based on a group of otherwise healthy people. The values in between those limits may depend on such factors as age, sex, and specimen type (blood, urine, spinal fluid, etc.) and can also be influenced by circumstantial situations such as fasting and exercise. While this site can help you understand some of the implications of your test results, the best source of this information is your healthcare provider. You can use what you learn about your results from Lab Tests Online to talk to your provider, be prepared to ask the right questions during that conversation, and to take an active role in your healthcare decisions.

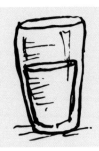

Drink plenty of water an hour before your test. Also, carry a snack bar or piece of fruit to eat after your blood draw. Most tests require a 12 hour fast. – Debra Raybern

The following ranges are considered normal for healthy adults. One of the columns in this blood work assessment chart asks you to list the body system. It is very important to know the body system most effected in your particular diagnosis, symptoms, or syndrome. Also, this helps you to narrow the focus of your eating plan; be careful to choose foods that support that system and avoid foods that are detrimental, as well as the supplements you will choose in a later step. Some issues naturally point to an organ or system, like fatty liver and kidney stones. Other names are not as straight forward, so you do not have an immediate place to target. This is where the assessments come in handy and allow you to pinpoint your starting point.

Input your result for each test in the second column. After you learn about supplements and essential oils in STEPS FIVE and SIX respectively, we will prompt you to return to this section and record the products you will use in the sixth column.

Test/ Determination	Your Result	Optimal Range	Test Guide	System of the Body	Natural Supplements and/or Essential Oils (see charts in STEPS FIVE and SIX)
Glucose/ Pancreas		70-110 mg/dL	Measures blood sugar levels.	Circulatory and Immune	
Fructosamine		1.20-1.60 mmol/L	A1c testing monitors glucose over a long period of time.	Circulatory Immune	
Blood urea nitrogen (BUN)		6-25 mg/dL	A by-product of protein metabolism and cleared by kidneys	Circulatory and Endocrine	
Creatine		0.60-1.50 mg/dL	A by-product of muscle metabolism cleared by kidneys. Protein diets may cause mild elevations.	Circulatory and Endocrine	
Alkaline phosphatase		30-115 U/L	Enzyme found primarily in the bone and liver. Due to its importance in bone-making progress, usually higher in children than adults. Pregnancy may elevate levels at times.	Circulatory, Skeletal, and Endocrine	

Total bilirubin		0.10-1.20 mg/dL	A by-product of the breakdown of old red blood cells and made into a water soluble form in the liver.	Circulatory and Endocrine	
SGOT (AST)		0-33 U/L	Enzyme from three main sources: skeletal muscle, heart muscle, and liver tissue. Certain medications or liver disorders may increase elevation.	Circulatory, Skeletal, Muscular, Immune, and Endocrine	
SGPT or ALT (Serum Glutamic-Pyruvic Transaminase or alanine aminotransferase)		7-35 U/L or 0.12–0.60 mckat/L for females 10-40 units per liter (U/L) or 0.17-0.68 microkatals per liter (mckat/L) for males	Used to screen for damage to or disease in the liver.	Circulatory and Endocrine	
Iron, Serum		Shown as low, normal, or high	Used to assess how much iron is being carried in the blood.	Circulatory and Immune	
Gama Glutamyltransferase		2-65 U/L	A liver enzyme present in various tissues.	Circulatory and Endocrine	
Total Protein		6.0-8.5 g/dL	Low values may be associated with peripheral edema or malnutrition. High values may suggest dehydration or chronic inflammation.	Circulatory and Digestion	

Total Cholesterol		Less than 200mg/dL	The measure of the total amount of cholesterol in your blood, including low-density lipoprotein (LDL) cholesterol and high-density lipoprotein (HDL) cholesterol.	Circulatory and Endocrine	
LDL		Less than 100mg/dL	Low-density lipoprotein, or bad cholesterol, the main source of cholesterol buildup and blockage in the arteries.	Circulatory and Endocrine	
HDL		60 mg/dL and higher	High-density lipoprotein cholesterol or good cholesterol helps remove cholesterol from your arteries.	Circulatory and Endocrine	
White Blood Count or WBC (Leukocyte Count; White Count)		4,500-11,000 white blood cells per microliter	Included in complete blood count (CBC), totals the number of white blood cells in a sample and often used in the general evaluation of a person's health.	Circulatory, Endocrine, and Immune	
Red Blood Count or RBD (Erythrocyte Count; Red Count)		$4.5\text{-}5.1 \times 10^6$ microliter for females

$4.5\text{-}5.9 \times 106/$ microliter for males | May be used to detect a problem with red blood cell production and/or lifespan | Circulatory, Endocrine, and Immune | |
| TSH – Thyroid Stimulating Hormone or Serum thyrotropin | | 0.4–4.2 microunits per milliliter (mcU/mL) or 0.4–4.2 milliunits per liter (mU/L) | Produced by the pituitary gland, which signals the thyroid gland to make and release thyroid hormones into the blood. | Circulatory and Endocrine | |

T3 or Serum Triiodothyronine		80-180 ng/dL	T3 is produced by the thyroid. Used to evaluate thyroid function.	Circulatory and Endocrine	
T4 or Serum thyroxine		4.6-12 ug/dL	T3 is produced by the thyroid. Used to evaluate thyroid function.	Circulatory and Endocrine	
Triglycerides		149 mg/dL or lower	Another form of fat in your blood that can raise your risk for heart disease.	Circulatory and Digestion	

Now that you have your test results and have listed your initial results in the chart above, use a highlighter to mark any items out of optimal range. Research this area and find out what nutritional, supplement, and/or lifestyle changes can bring this number into range. Then, as you have future tests you can record the values in this chart below, which will provide a great picture of your improved wellness over the long term. The example below will show you to fill in the blanks.

Test	Optimal Range	7/15/16	12/1/16	7/1/17	7/1/18	7/1/19
Glucose/ Pancreas	70-110 mg/dL	115	107	98	93	84
Fructosamine	1.20-1.60 mmol/L	1.60	1.43	1.37	1.37	1.3
Blood urea nitrogen (BUN)	6-25 mg/dL	24	24	23	18	15

Test	Optimal Range					
Glucose/Pancreas	70-110 mg/dL					
Fructosamine	1.20-1.60 mmol/L					
Blood urea nitrogen (BUN)	6-25 mg/dL					
Creatine	0.60-1.50 mg/dL					
Alkaline phosphatase	30-115 U/L					
Total bilirubin	0.10-1.20 mg/dL					
SGOT (AST)	0-33 U/L					
SGPT (ALT)	25					
Iron, Serum	100					
Gama Glutamyltransferase	2-65 U/L					
Total Protein	6.0-8.5 g/dL					

Total Cholesterol	180-220					
LDL	Less than 100mg/dL					
HDL	60 mg/dL and higher					
WBC White Blood Count	4,500-11,000 white blood cells per microliter (mcL)					
RBD Red Blood Count	4.5-5.1 x 106 microliter for females 4.5-5.9 x 106/ microliter for males					
TSH – Thyroid Stimulating Hormone	0.4-4.2 microunits per milliliter (mcU/mL) or 0.4-4.2 milliunits per liter (mU/L)					
T3	80-180 ng/dL					
T4	4.6-12 ug/dL					
Triglycerides	149 mg/dL or lower					

In the chart below, list of all the medications you take and why. We provided an example on the first line.

Medicine	Why	Body System(s)	Date Began	Date Ended
Cholesterol/Lipitor	Elevated bad cholesterol levels	Cardiovascular	January 2015	February 2017

Now, make a list of all the symptoms that chronically bother you and the organ or body system with which it is associated. You will want to note the length of time you have experienced each issue and prioritize which ones you will work on first. You may not know of the natural solution just yet so that can be added later.

Please realize that an issue you have had for 10 years may not be as easily brought back into balance as one you've only had a few months. So, even though you'd like to make it a top priority, it will better serve you to first tackle an issue that cleansing, nourishing, and a few well-placed oils and supplements can help. When it comes off the list, it will boost your confidence and help you jump into tackling the next challenge.

For some of you, there will be issues that you have dealt with for a long time, and for some of you these may be serious. It may take longer for your body to repair and restore, but don't give up! Your body was fearfully and wonderfully made!

> Do you believe whole heartedly that GOD designed your body to heal itself, given the right nutrients and support? Your belief will be directly related to your success, so once you believe change is possible you can align your actions and progress! – Laura Hopkins

To find nutrients that support each body system and the foods they are found in, please refer to *Nutrition 101: Choose Life!*, a book we co-authored from growinghealthyhomes.com.

In STEPS FOUR, FIVE, and SIX, you will learn more about body system solutions.

The chart below requires you to research supplements, foods, and nutrients to support specific body systems. You can find such information in *Nutrition 101: Choose Life!*, the Young Living reference guides, and other reference books.

Health Goals			
Challenge	**Body System Affected**	**How long/Priority**	**Solutions**
Cholesterol	Cardiovascular, Endocrine (Liver)	5 years, low	Diet, NingXia Red®, Liver Detox

If unhealthy has become your body's natural state, then it may seem to resist healthy changes. However, the body is actually healing. German physician and the father of American homeopathy, Constantine Hering observed how the body responded during the healing process and summarized the process into the following laws:
- The body seeks to externalize disease or remove it when allowed.
- Symptoms will appear and disappear in the reverse order of their appearance upon the body. Allopathic medicine refers to this process as a "Herxheimer Reaction."
- The body heals from top to bottom, from within outwards, from more vital organs to less vital organs, and in reverse order of their appearance.

Symptoms will likely surface as part of the healing process. There are natural products that help alleviate some of the discomfort associated with healing. In the STEP FOUR about Cleansing, you will learn more about these. However, learning to accept the process and stay committed to your plan is your most valuable asset.

Please read this carefully:

While the authors have taken charge of their wellness, along with millions of other people around the world, please don't ignore an issue or system. If you are not willing to do the research and the work to reach your own healthy best, then take your medicine. Remember to work with your doctor as much as you can. This manual was not written to encourage you to ignoring a health issue. You must learn to listen to your body and help it be in its best possible shape.

> If these symptoms get to be too much for you, back off or slow down a little. Then, reassess what you can do and return to the program as soon as possible. Should you push through? Listen to your body. If you have time to rest and add nightly detox baths to aid in the process, it will greatly help. – Debra Raybern

Detoxifying Bath Soak
- 1/2 cup Dead Sea salts
- 5 drops Grapefruit essential oil
- 5 drops of body system specific oil (such as JuvaFlex® for kidney, Peppermint for digestion)
- 1/2 cup bentonite clay

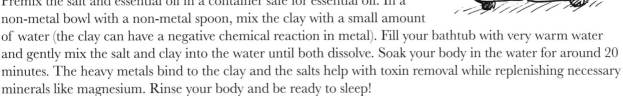

Premix the salt and essential oil in a container safe for essential oil. In a non-metal bowl with a non-metal spoon, mix the clay with a small amount of water (the clay can have a negative chemical reaction in metal). Fill your bathtub with very warm water and gently mix the salt and clay into the water until both dissolve. Soak your body in the water for around 20 minutes. The heavy metals bind to the clay and the salts help with toxin removal while replenishing necessary minerals like magnesium. Rinse your body and be ready to sleep!

> After bathing, use Genesis™ Body Lotion or Cel-Lite Magic™ Massage Oil to soothe the skin and aid circulation. I love to use Detoxzyme® and Sulfurzyme® to help minimize any negative responses to detoxification. – Laura Hopkins

Oxygen

"All the while my breath is in me, and the spirit of God is in my nostrils." – Job 27:3

None of us have to think about breathing to accomplish this natural and necessary task. However, proper breathing is essential to your physical, mental, and spiritual health. It not only improves metabolism, but it also helps relieve stress. Here are the simple steps for intentional breathing that can make a big difference in your day.

1. Inhale through your nose for four seconds. Your abdomen should expand.

2. Hold the air in your lungs for four seconds.

3. Exhale through your nose for four seconds, expelling all of the air. Your abdomen should return to normal.

4. Repeat as necessary.

Why the nose? Among other things, breathing through the nose exercises the diaphragm and directs oxygen to all five lobes of the lungs rather than just two with mouth breathing.

Breathing is free and can be done anywhere. So, why not commit to being intentional about breathing?

Make a commitment to yourself and fill in the blanks below:

I will choose to take _____ intentional breaths at _____ in the morning, _____ in the afternoon, and _____ before bed.

Exercise

Aerobic Exercise, by definition, is the strengthening of the heart and lungs through oxygen usage during exercise. This includes endurance activities that increase heart rate like walking, cycling, running, and rowing.

Anaerobic Exercise is short exertion, high-intensity movement like jumping (rope), sprinting (short distances), or weightlifting.

> I love the challenge and comradery of CrossFit! At first, I was intimidated by the thought of just stepping foot in the gym, but I love that it's family friendly and adaptable for each person. Because they change up the workouts to target various areas and focus on high intensity interval training, anyone can do it and at their own ability level. My goal is to have long, lean muscles, not to be bulky, so I focus on lighter weights with more repetition. – Laura Hopkins

Depending on your level of fitness, you may have shortness of breath when you begin. Please consult with your health care provider to be sure you are attempting exercise within your current fitness level. Slow and steady wins the race. You can work up to a greater fitness level a little at a time. Start where you are comfortable and maintain the consistency to build your stamina and endurance. Active parents create healthy habits for their children by involving the whole family exercising.

Can you …

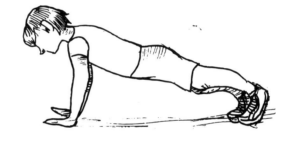

Touch your toes?

Walk in place for one minute?

Do a push-up?

Climb stairs with ease?

Jog to the mailbox?

Learning your capabilities and limits will help you set realistic goals. Do you want to be active enough to play with your children and grandchildren, or do you want to train for a triathlon? What do you want to accomplish through regular exercise? Record your thoughts below. Use this as the brainstorming portion for the first question on MY PLAN ("I choose to exercise because")

_____

_____

_____

_____

_____

_____

Stretching

Stretching is natural and necessary for flexibility. Injuries often occur if we skip stretching, stretch incorrectly, or at the wrong time. It's best to warm the muscles slightly before engaging in stretches with three to five minutes of a light aerobic warm-up. Then, use a combination of both static and dynamic stretching as described below.

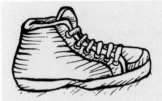

Will you be tying your own shoes at age 80 because you have continued with exercise and stretching to remain flexible or will someone else be doing that task for you? – Debra Raybern

Static Stretching is when you hold a stretch in a challenging but comfortable position for a period of time for 10 to 30 seconds. Examples include standing or sitting to touch your toes, pulling your knees to your chest, or intertwining your fingers and pushing your palms over your head.

Dynamic Stretching is a controlled, smooth, and deliberate stretch through movement in comfortable range of motion repeatedly, usually 10 to 12 times. A few examples include lunges, arm circles, and leg swings.

Excuse-busters:

- If you prefer to exercise in a group, join a local Curves, Boot Camp, or CrossFit in your community. Gym memberships also usually include weekly classes.
- If you prefer to exercise by yourself, join a gym or find community resources (running trails, equipment)
- If you cannot leave your house to exercise, there are hundreds of online or DVD resources.
- If you do have time to exercise, you just need to schedule it.
- I think it might be better to say – If you are not yet disciplined with your exercise, schedule it on your calendar or planner so it becomes an appointment for wellness.
- Do not allow excuses or other people to impede your desire to live a full vibrant and healthy life.

It's easy to hit snooze on the alarm or even avoid exercise at the end of the day. If you don't have a plan, it is easier to let excuses keep you from taking care of yourself. Create a plan, block out this time on your calendar just as you would another important appointment, and find accountability. Even if you don't have a workout partner, tell someone what you're doing and ask that person to keep you accountable to your goals. Children are especially good accountability and exercise partners. What are some activities you can do together with your family that will benefit everyone and involve quality time too? List your favorites below:

_____

_____

_____

_____

Exercise Equipment

STOP! Before you go buy expensive, bulky exercise equipment you may bring home and only use for a week before storing it under the bed or in the garage, test them out at the local gym. Hold off on your big ticket purchase until you have spent several months establishing exercise as a habit and know that you are self-motivated enough to use this home equipment daily or multiple times a week.

One way to keep yourself accountable and keep you active is to use a fitness tracker. If they help you be a better you, then the cost is well worth it. If interested, check out these: Apple Watch, Fit Bit, or Garmin for wrist worn trackers. Remember to be careful of electromagnetic frequencies. We will discuss this more in STEP TWO.

Whew!
- ❏ Assessments and evaluations done!
- ❏ Areas of focus identified, check.
- ❏ On to STEP TWO

Just Between Us Girls

It's no secret there is a definite difference between the male and female bodies. Talking about those differences alone would require a separate book, so we will just stick with those normal and natural changes – and the symptoms that go with them – that occur in a woman's body from puberty to menopause.

Nearly every magazine or book on women's health, health food stores, and all your female friends will have their opinions on how you can manage these occasional symptoms, but it may boil down to just one organ: the liver.

You can take all kinds of supplements to assist in balancing your hormone levels at any age, but many do not realize the role the liver plays in hormonal health. It is the liver's job to process – not create – estrogen. Too little or too much estrogen can cause a myriad of problems, starting in puberty and lasting through childbearing years. Some ladies will experience fibroids, endometriosis, painful menses, irregular cycles, cysts, heavy bleeding, and more. Most of these are due in large part to excessive estrogen.

By the time most women enter into menopause and estrogen slows down, they have too little estrogen and symptoms of menopause such as hot flashes, dryness, loss of bone strength, and challenges with the heart, skin, and hair come into play.

What if during this Road to Wellness journey, you took a little extra time and concentrated on cleansing the liver and supporting it with a couple of perfect foods to help keep your estrogen imbalance?

People get excess estrogen, not because the body makes it, but from the foods we eat, the water we drink, the air we breathe, and the products we use. These estrogens are called xenoestrogens. They mimic the body's own estrogen and block it from being used properly. Then, this excess estrogen finds its way to organs like the uterus and begins to accelerate tissue growth, often leading to fibroids.

As we cleanse the liver, we are not removing estrogen. We are allowing the liver to process estrogen in order for the body to receive the real and proper amounts, sending them where they're supposed to go, and allowing the xenoestrogens to be removed from the body.

When I was consulting, young girls and ladies tried various supplements –many specific for the issues they were addressing – and many times they were quite successful. However, nearly every single time a woman went on a liver cleanse prior to taking supplements, those supplements were never needed. Fibroids vanished, periods returned to normal, hot flashes ceased, and life in general went back to normal. There is no reason that a woman at any age needs to suffer when a really good liver cleanse can provide so much relief. This does not mean that a supplement won't be of great value, but until you address the liver, you will not get your maximum benefit. – Debra Raybern

The other item that's extremely important to female hormonal health is actually a food.

It doesn't matter how you eat it: steamed, sautéed, juiced, raw, dunked in ranch dressing, sliced, shredded, or chopped – this food is paramount to your body handling estrogen.

Can you guess what food it is? Broccoli!

Why broccoli? Because it contains the substance DIM, which stands for Diindoylymethane and is also found in lesser amounts in cauliflower, kale, bok choy, Brussels sprouts, and cabbage. For those of you who have been told to stay away from some of these foods as they may affect the function of the thyroid gland, there's no need to do so completely, but you will want to just lightly steam them to prevent that effect.

Because this simple system has such great and profound results, please take time to review the various liver cleansing options in STEP FOUR and pick one for every month this year, including the coffee enema or colonic (also in STEP FOUR) and see what a difference they make. Then, as you continue to supplement, you'll see that less is required. From the start of menses in puberty through the golden years of menopause, you will not be nagged by what others consider the normal concerns that take up a great deal of our life.

Does this seem like too simple of a solution to your ongoing problems? Well, maybe it does, but that's how God made our bodies.

Keep it cleansed, keep it nourished, and it has the power to heal itself.

My Plan

Copy this sentence in the space below and say it out loud:

"I desire to be well and thrive in life."

_____

❏ I have completed the assessment phase and recorded my results.

❏ I have identified my health goals and chosen a starting point.

I will choose to take _____ intentional breaths at _____ in the morning, _____ in the afternoon, and _____ before bed.

I choose to exercise because:

_____

I commit to being active _____ minutes a day and _____ times a week.

I will exercise at _____ a.m./p.m. with _____

I will exercise at _____ a.m./p.m. with _____

I will exercise at _____ a.m./p.m. with _____

I will exercise at _____ a.m./p.m. with _____

I will exercise at _____ a.m./p.m. with _____

Aerobic Warm-ups I will do:

_____

Dynamic Stretches I will do:

_____

Exercise I will do:

_____

My accountability partner(s) is/are:

_____

STEP TWO
Prepare the Environment

STEP TWO
Prepare the Environment

"A journey of a thousand miles begins with a single step." – Lao Tzu

There's no denying it; we live in a toxic world. The air, food, water, and the environment at large is full of harmful toxins and chemicals. The war on health begins and is won on the home front. Man-made or synthesized chemicals on the market intended to clean our homes and bodies are wreaking havoc on our bodies, minds, and emotions. Taking the time to sweep your home of all potential hazards is both worthwhile and important for long term. This is especially true of chemicals that come in contact with the skin because it has no safeguards, and topically absorbed chemicals go directly into organs.

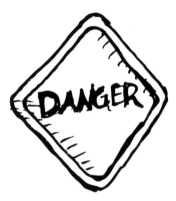

We understand it may be a little overwhelming to identify and replace these toxic products and cleanse the body down to the cellular level. This section will walk you through the process.

There are thousands of naturally occurring chemicals used in perfectly safe products. Just because you can't pronounce it doesn't mean it's not safe. However, just because the label says it's safe doesn't mean there aren't dangers hidden in the ingredient list. The authors recommend all of the recipes in Appendix S of *Nutrition 101: Choose Life!*, as well as the Chemical Free Home books with natural alternative recipes by Melissa Poepping, CNHP.

If you want to clean your house of dangerous chemicals, you must know their names, what they do, and where to look. The following list is an alphabetical, non-inclusive list that will jumpstart your research. Also, search for the Environmental Working Group's Guide to Healthy Cleaning.

Ammonia

Found In: Cleaners that shine bathroom fixtures, glass, sinks, and jewelry, and because of its high nitrogen content, it's also found in fertilizer.

Health Risks: Poisoning can occur from just breathing ammonia. Ammonia mixed with bleach will creates toxic chlorine gas, which can be deadly.

Healthier Choice: Vodka or witch hazel can produce the desired shine on metal or mirrored surfaces. Because both are alcohol based, they can dry without rinsing. They also clean mirrors, eyeglasses, jewelry, sinks, and certain floors and countertops.

Chlorine

Found In: Cleaners labeled for scouring, heavy-duty cleaners (toilet bowl, mildew removal, laundry whiteners), and in some communities' tap water.

Health Risks: The health risks from chlorine may be slow to surface and are typically chronic in nature; Concerns about endocrine disruption, specifically to the thyroid as it prevents the absorption of iodine and tyrosine.

Healthier Choice: For scrubbing, stick to baking soda and Thieves Household Cleaner. To reduce your exposure to chlorine through tap water, install filters on your faucets and showerheads or look into a whole-house filter.

Fluoride

Found In: tap water, toothpaste

Health Risks: As it occurs naturally in some water sources, up to two-thirds of Americans are exposed to tap water with fluoride. In most communities, pharmaceutical-grade fluoride is added to water to supposedly help prevent tooth decay and diminish cavities. However, this benefit has not been proven, and most European countries have refused to subject citizens to fluoridated water. The World Health Organization recommends fluoride levels in drinking water stay between 0.8 and 1.2 milligrams (mg) per liter and below 1.5 mg per liter.

Healthier Choice: Water filters, specifically whole-house filters, are the most effective method for cleaning the water coming into your home. These range in price, so many start with filtration systems for drinking water first; however, exposure to fluoride during bathing also should be considered. Adding the mineral selenium to the diet strengthens immunity; food sources include good quality tuna and salmon, asparagus, and eggs. Thieves® oral care products, including toothpaste, mouthwash, and dental floss, are an easy and necessary replacement as absorption in the mouth is one of the quickest ways toxins enter the bloodstream.

Glycol ethers

Found In: Window, kitchen, and multipurpose cleaners.

Health Risks: The most common offenders are 2-butoxyethanol (EGBE) and methoxydiglycol (DEGME). A product containing more than 12.5% EGBE is classed as a hazardous substance by the Australian Department of Health. Currently, U.S. law does not require it to be listed on a product's label, but the U.S. EPA sets a standard on EGBE for workplace safety. Most concerns are related to using the chemicals in contained areas without ventilation.

Healthier Choice: Newspaper and diluted vinegar or Thieves® Household Cleaner are perfect substitutes. Baking soda and essential oils also may be added for additional cleaning power and beneficial fragrance.

Perchloroethylene also known as "PERC"

Found In: Dry-cleaning solutions, spot removers, and carpet and upholstery cleaners.

Health Risks: A neurotoxin also classified by the U.S. EPA as a "possible carcinogen" because scientists still are learning the long-term effects of PFCs to the human body. The route of exposure is most often inhalation: that telltale smell on clothes when they return from the dry cleaner, or the fumes that linger after cleaning carpets.

Healthier Choice: Ask your dry cleaner if they offer water-based technology rather than chemical solvents. "Dry clean only" items can be taken to a "wet cleaner" instead. For a safer spot remover, look for a nontoxic brand at a natural market, or rub undiluted castile soap directly on stains before washing.

Perfluorochemicals (PFCs)

Found In: Non-stick cookware and stain-resistant coatings on clothing, furniture, and carpets.

Health Risks: PFCs are endocrine disruptors that are completely resistant to biodegradation – in the environment or in your body. Scientists are still learning the long-term effects on the human body, but animal studies have shown damage to the thyroid and sex hormone levels.

Healthier Choice: Choose ceramic, stainless steel, cast iron, or titanium cookware, and choose clothing fabric that is natural and chemical-free.

Phthalates

Found In: Fragranced household products, such as air fresheners, soap, paper products, and plastic food containers (recycling label 3). Watch for the word "fragrance" on a label because that most likely means phthalates are present.

Health Risks: Known endocrine disruptors.

Healthier Choice: Choose fragrance-free or all-natural organic products. Avoid aerosol or plug-in air fresheners, and use diffusers with essential oils instead. Air out rooms by opening windows when possible.

Propylene Glycol

Found In: Personal care products such as shampoo, toothpaste, shaving foam, body washes, and facial cleansers, and food products

Health Risks: European authorities have limited use of propylene glycol to mostly non-food uses. Various research and studies raise concern for the skin, liver, kidney, and cell mutations following contact with propylene glycol.

Healthier Choice: Use sulfate-free products for washing your body, and nourishing and hydrating the skin. Young Living Essential Oils offers a multitude of options infused with oils and natural products.

Quaternary Ammonium Compounds or "Quats"

Found In: Fabric softener liquids and sheets; most household cleaners labeled "antibacterial."

Health Risks: An antimicrobial that breeds antibiotic-resistant bacteria, and a skin irritant linked to dermatitis and potentially to respiratory issues.

Healthier Choice: White vinegar added to the rinse cycle works just as well as fabric softener and soap residue remover. Wool dryer balls can replace dryer sheets used to eliminate static cling. Thieves® Household Cleaner (dilute as directed on the bottle) is effective for all household needs.

Sodium Hydroxide (NaOH)

Found In: Oven cleaners and drain openers

Health Risks: Lye or caustic soda, as it is commonly known, can cause severe burns if it touches your skin, gets in your eyes, or you inhale it.

Healthier Choice: You can clean the grimiest oven with Thieves® Household Cleaner and baking soda. Granted, it takes longer and potentially some elbow grease, but For drains, use a mechanical "snake" tool or enlist this natural clog remedy from the Green Living Ideas Web site: "Pour a cup of baking soda and a cup of vinegar down the drain and plug it for 30 minutes. After the bubbles die down, run hot water down the drain to clear the debris."

Sulfate compounds (sulfates)

Found In: Personal care products such as shampoo, toothpaste, shaving foam, body washes, and facial cleansers. They are listed under a myriad of names, the most common being Sodium Lauryl Sulfate (SLS), Sodium Laureth Sulfate (SLES), Sodium Lauryl Sulfoacetate, Sodium Lauroyl Isoethionate, Sodium Lauroyl Taurate, Sodium Cocoyl Isoethionate, Sodium Lauroyl Methyl Isoethionate, Sodium Lauroyl Sarcosinate, and Disodium Laureth Sulfosuccinate.

Health Risks: Sulfates disrupt the natural biome of our bodies. They are primarily surfactants, which foam and are the reason why we associate clean with foaming or bubbles. In addition to cleaning away dirt and grease, sulfates also strip skin of vital moisture, peptides, proteins and water-proofing oils, and expose it to harmful elements.

Healthier Choice: Use sulfate-free products for washing your body and nourishing and hydrating the skin. Young Living Essential Oils offers a multitude of options infused with oils and natural products.

Triclosan

Found In: "Antibacterial" soaps, hand sanitizers, clothing, furniture, and toys

Health Risks: May disrupt endocrine system; possible carcinogen. Regulated by the EPA as a pesticide. Because concentrations of triclosan found in rivers and streams are contaminating wildlife and there was no evidence to prove these antibacterial products were effective, they're no longer allowed to be marketed, but still remain in many products sold before the ban in September 2016.

Healthier Choice: Washing with water and good-quality soap, like Thieves® Foaming Hand Soap, Hand Sanitizer, and Dishwashing Liquid.

Out With the Bad, in With the Clean!

Now that you have removed toxic items from the home, here are some natural, effective replacements that you can use to create a clean environment that benefits your health! Use the following checklists to assist you with toxin removal and replacement.

> Keep in mind that many cleaners packaged or marketed as "green" contain toxins that are not good for people or pets. Also, many cleaners that are completely natural and safe cannot effectively combat microbials in your environment. You must choose wisely! – Laura Hopkins

While there are many green cleaners on the market, the authors prefer Thieves® products because they effectively clean and rid a home or microorganisms, and they are safe for every member of the family, including babies, the elderly, and pets. Thieves® Household Cleaner is a general household cleaning alternative for countertops, walls, floors, bath tubs, toilets, windows, and just about anything that needs cleaning. The cleaner comes highly concentrated, so follow the dilution recommendations on the back.

Other products include Thieves® Spray, Thieves® Hand Purifier, Thieves® Laundry Soap, Thieves® Foaming Hand Soap, Thieves® Fruit and Veggie Wash and Spray, and Thieves® Dishwashing Liquid.

Additionally, there are numerous products for oral, skin, beauty, and hair care and maintenance. Diffusing essential oils is also a significant method of refreshing and cleansing your home; feel free to experiment with combinations of singles oils or blends that you already enjoy. Review the Young Living product guide to find more solutions.

DIY recipes

Spot Remover
    2 Tbsp. cream of tartar
    2 drops eucalyptus or lemon essential oil

Add a little water to make a paste and spread over the stain. Apply immediately for best results. Allow to dry before washing.

Abrasive Cleaner – great for sinks, bathtubs, and showers!
    1 cup each of cheap table salt, borax, and baking soda (large boxes are found in the laundry aisle)
    20 total drops of either Purification®, Lemon, or Thieves® essential oil.

Place in a sealed glass jar and shake into surfaces when needed.

Chrome, stainless steel, copper, and tin polish
    1 Tbsp. of baking soda
    1 drop of lemon oil

Rub on surfaces with a soft, damp cloth and the rinse with warm water. Dry with a separate cloth.

Sachets for storage – protect your winter items without the chemicals of mothballs

Fill small cotton muslin bags with cedar shavings and mixed with a sprinkling of any of the following eucalyptus radiata, patchouli, peppermint, Purification® or RepelAroma™ essential oil (animal scents collection). Place the sachets in closets, drawers, or storage containers.

KITCHEN	Product(s) found	Replaced with
Ammonia		
Chlorine		
Fluoride		
Glycol ethers		
PERC		
PFCs		
Phthalates		
Propylene glycol		
Quats		
NaOH		
Sulfates		
Triclosan		

BATHROOMS	Product(s) found	Replaced with
Ammonia		
Chlorine		
Fluoride		
Glycol ethers		
PERC		
PFCs		
Phthalates		
Propylene glycol		
Quats		
NaOH		
Sulfates		
Triclosan		

LAUNDRY ROOM/MUDROOM	Product(s) found	Replaced with
Ammonia		
Chlorine		
Glycol ethers		
PERC		
PFCs		
Phthalates		

Propylene glycol		
Quats		
NaOH		
Sulfates		
Triclosan		

BEDROOMS		
	Product(s) found	**Replaced with**
Ammonia		
Chlorine		
Glycol ethers		
PERC		
PFCs		
Phthalates		
Propylene glycol		
Quats		
NaOH		
Sulfates		
Triclosan		

GARAGE		
	Product(s) found	**Replaced with**
Ammonia		
Chlorine		
Glycol ethers		
PERC		
PFCs		
Phthalates		
Propylene glycol		
Quats		
NaOH		
Sulfates		
Triclosan		

My Plan

Copy this sentence in the space below and say it out loud.

"I desire to be well and thrive in life."

_____

I am committed to being a conscientious consumer and find or make natural cleaners and products that keep my home free of toxins.

I found _____ chemicals in _____ rooms of my home; I will replace these chemicals with healthy, natural versions.

(Use your lists above to keep track of what you are replacing.)

My accountability partner(s) is/are:

_____

For additional accountability, you may choose to publicly post before and after photos of the products you are discarding and the new safer, people, pet and environment friendly alternatives on your social media accounts.

STEP THREE
Determining What's Fuel and What's Not

STEP THREE
Determining What's Fuel and What's Not

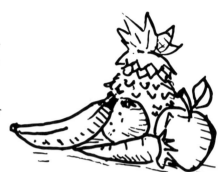

Each person has the ability to change their health by changing their diet. In the curriculum we co-authored *Nutrition 101: Choose Life!*, we discussed how we're fearfully and wonderfully made and how food affects our bodies, both good and bad ways. Most people would focus on weight loss when thinking of food, but a number on a scale does not reflect your overall health. Specific strategies for weight management are listed on page 89.

With so many nutritional lifestyle choices, it's hard to understand what they all mean and intend to do. Let's take a look at some of the most popular and break down what they do and don't do.

Lifestyle Nutrition

Autoimmune Protocol (AIP) or the Paleo Approach
A spin-off of the original Paleo program, AIP is specific to those with autoimmune disease, which is any disease where the body fights against itself. AIP food choices work to reduce inflammation in the intestines and promote those tissues to heal themselves. Specifically, it is geared toward healing the mucosal lining of the intestines and lowering overall body tissue inflammation. Inflammation is often the beginning of a flare up for those with autoimmune challenges.

Resources and Recipes: autoimmune-paleo.com, grazedandenthused.com/autoimmuneprotocolrecipes

Dairy free
Milk contains lactase, a sugar, that must be broken down by lactose, the enzyme that helps the human body digest food. Those who choose this lifestyle can choose to eat vegan cheeses and other modified products made from nuts and plants.

Resources and Recipes: vegan.com/dairy-free, myhdiet.com/Fall-In-Love-With-Food-Again/

Gluten-free
Originally developed to treat Celiac disease by eliminating the cause of inflammation in the small intestines, a gluten-free lifestyle excludes gluten protein from the diet and personal care products. Gluten is naturally found in grains such as wheat, barley, rye, and triticale, a cross between wheat and rye. Oat, rice, corn, quinoa, almond, and other flours without gluten are commonly used as substitutes in recipes. Those who choose to avoid gluten may not be diagnosed with Celiac disease, but still have sensitivities. Non-genetically modified gluten, such as that in Young Living's einkorn products, seems to be less of an issue with this group of people.

Resources and Recipes: glutenfreeliving.com/gluten-free-foods/diet/basic-diet/, elanaspantry.com/diets/gluten-free/

Macrobiotic
Taken from the Greek "macro" for great and "bios" for life, using macrobiotic principles means to determine the foods best suited to a person based on their current condition and what he or she wants to become. This system allows one to learn to live within the natural order of life, the constantly changing nature of all things.

What works for one, may not necessarily work for another and what works today may not work the next. To achieve a macrobiotic lifestyle requires a shift in thinking from a static view of life to a dynamic and flexible one.

Resources and Recipes: ohsawamacrobiotics.com/macrobiotics/what-is-macrobiotics

Mucusless
Based on the theory that we should not add mucus into the body faster than it can be eliminated, this low-mucus, preventative lifestyle is designed to benefit the respiratory system and also catarrh, the constipating mucus, in body tissues from head to toe. In addition to meeting the parameters of a vegan lifestyle, it also eliminates all sugar products, flour, and conventional salt.

Resources and Recipes: healthfree.com/view_newsletter.php?id=157&, mucusfreelife.com/mucusless-diet-food-list/

Paleo
Named for the Paleolithic period, during which, evolutionists believe man was a pre-agricultural, hunter-gatherer, this lifestyle focuses on grass-produced meats, fish/seafood, fresh fruits and veggies, eggs, nuts and seeds, and healthful oils such as olive, walnut, flaxseed, macadamia, avocado, coconut. Flours made from almond and coconut are common recipe replacements.

Resources and Recipes: authoritynutrition.com/paleo-diet-meal-plan-and-menu/, Paleogrubs.com

FODMAP
Short for Fermentable Oligo-, Di-, Monosaccharides, and Polyols, this diet often is used by people with irritable bowel disorders or other symptoms stemming from inflammatory bowel disease. This diet restricts fructose (fruits, high fructose corn syrup, honey; lactose (dairy); fructans also known as inulins (wheat, garlic, onions); galactans (beans, lentils, legumes); and polyols (sorbitol, mannitol, xylitol, fruits containing stones such as cherries, avocado, peaches, etc).

Resources and Recipes: fodmapliving.com

Ketogenic
Designed as a therapeutic diet for children with epilepsy, the ketogenic way of eating encourages consumption of high amounts of fat and minimal amounts of protein and carbohydrates for healthy body growth and repair. Sufficient calories are necessary for the body to maintain adequate weight for the person's height and age; this system encourages a 4:1 ratio by weight of fat to proteins and carbohydrates.

Resources and Recipes: ketogenic-diet-resource.com/ketogenic-diet-plan.html

Vegetarian/Vegan
While all vegetarian lifestyles focus on consuming fruits, vegetables, legumes, grains, seeds, and nuts, traditional vegetarians do not eat meat, but may eat products from animals like dairy or eggs. Lactovegetarians do not consume dairy products. Ovolactarians do not eat eggs. Semi-vegetarians do not eat red meat, but consume chicken, fish and products from animals. Vegan diets eliminate all meat, animal products, and even products like honey because it is made by bees. As more and more people are reducing or eliminating grains from their diets, look at quinoa, rice or almond flour or very-low gluten Einkorn pastas and flour.

Resources and Recipes: mayoclinic.org/healthy-lifestyle/nutrition-and-healthy-eating/in-depth/vegetarian-diet/art-20046446, myhdiet.com/Fall-In-Love-With-Food-Again/

Whole 30

With an emphasis on developing a healthy metabolism, reducing systemic inflammation, and discovering how foods impact the human body, this initial 30-day program allows consumption of meat, seafood, eggs, vegetables, some fruit, and fats from fruits, oils, nuts and seeds. The purpose is to eat foods with ingredients one can pronounce or no ingredients at all. For the first 30 days, completely avoid sugar, alcohol, grains, legumes, dairy, carrageenan, MSG, sulfites, or healthy "junk food" to replace what you ate on the Standard American Diet. Ultimately, the 30-days are intended to extend to healthy, long-term lifestyle changes.

Resources and Recipes: whole30.com/whole30-program-rules/

Blood Type Programs

Eating according to your blood type was made popular from the work of Dr. J. D'Adamo, shared in his best-selling book, *Eat Right for Your Blood Type*. He explains that just as our fingerprints are unique, so are the bio-markers in our blood. With each drop of blood and all other body tissues, these antigens influence how your body reacts to the food you eat. When a certain food binds to your blood type antigen, it can trigger fatigue, headaches, digestive and skin issues, and unwanted weight gain or loss.

Resources and Recipes: dadamo.com

Body Type Programs

There has been much said about the value of understanding your body type in order to know the foods that benefit your health and weight. Several styles of diets for various body types exist; some have three types, but most have four. The theory fueling these programs is that we all are born with a dominant gland that influences our body's biochemical functioning and determines differences in body chemistry balance, metabolic function, and energy usage.

Resources and Recipes: precisionnutrition.com/all-about-body-type-eating, thedietcentre.com.sg/services/body-typing-body-composition.html

The basic four types are PARA, ESTRO, SUPRA, and NEURO. Some authors take these four basic types and expand them to include combination types. Body Type information is easily found on the internet, including the recommended food choices for each type. Though these lists include the foods a body type is drawn to, these are not the foods that benefit their overall wellbeing, and in most cases, would be avoided or limited.

The PARA type is a person with a straight-up-and-down physique without much of a waist who tends to gain weight all over. They mostly crave carbohydrates and sugars. A PARA body type often has an over-stimulated thyroid (which can be either hypo or hyperthyroid). The PARA type belongs to that part of the endocrine system most stimulated by sugars and carbohydrates.

The ESTRO type relates to that part of the endocrine system – the gonadal system or sex glands – a major gland of the endocrine system. ESTROs are most stimulated by spicy, fried, and fatty foods high in salt content. Their build is generally characterized by smaller shoulders, wider hips, and larger thighs.

The NEURO type connects to the part of the endocrine systems most stimulated by dairy and fatty foods – the nerve and pituitary glands. Information concerned with the well-being of an individual and gathered by the nervous system is transmitted by the hypothalamus, which regulates secretion of pituitary hormones. The classic NEURO shape is lean and thin, like a skinny version of the PARA shape.

The SUPRA type belongs to that part of the endocrine system – the suprarenal gland – a major gland of the endocrine system, and they are most stimulated by proteins. Think of this person as having broad shoulders and small hips. Professional swimmers and body builders often exhibit this type.

In Summary

You don't have to just pick one and stick with it forever. There may be times when you want to eat an all raw or vegan diet for a few weeks, possibly as a precursor to a longer cleanse. Why not try each of these for a couple weeks to a month and see how your body responds?

Please note that any time the body abruptly changes from one eating style to another, there will be changes, including some detoxification simply because you are now eating in a way that requires different digestion and elimination. Remember, just because a friend, book, or website may tout the virtues of the plan they are advocating, it does not mean it is necessarily right for you. Feel free to experiment, maybe even combine what you experience as the best of several plans, and always remember it's okay to make a change down the road.

So, which of these lifestyles or another healthy lifestyle appeals to you?

_____

Which plan will you try first?

_____

Once you commit to taking healthy steps, you will need to equip yourself with training, tips, and tools to choose and prepare the best fuel for your body. Consider it a kitchen makeover and you are the contractor! During this step, you are going to RID your home of toxins and junk and replenish your shelves and cupboards with food that heals and brings life. You may also need to add a few kitchen tools like a blender, a good set of knives, or a juicer. We will share our favorites at the end of this chapter.

Be a Label Reader

When you select food, be sure to look at the list of ingredients and scan the nutritional information. The fewer ingredients listed, the better, and the ingredients should be recognizable from real-food sources. Watch for products with sugar listed as the first or second ingredient; you'll be surprised that most products, even non-sugary foods, contain sugar as a top ingredient. Words ending in -ol are sugars.

Rid

Choose a time when you can go through each area (refrigerator, pantry/cupboards, and freezer) without interruption. Below is an alphabetical list of some of the worst offenders of food additives.

- Aluminum additives

- Artificial colors or flavors

- Artificial sweeteners (Aspartame, Acesulfame-K/Acesulfame Potassium, Cyclamates, Saccharine, and Sucralose.)

- Preservatives (Butylated Hydroxyanisole aka BHA, Butylated Hydroxyltoluene aka BHT, or Tertiary butylhydroquinone aka TBHQ

- Diacetyl

- High Fructose Corn Syrup or corn syrup

- Hydrogenated and partially hydrogenated fat

- Manufactured oils (*Canola oil, vegetable oil, or cottonseed oil*)

- Monosodium Glutamate (MSG) (May be listed as glutamic acid, glutamate, monopotassium glutamate, yeast extract, anything "hydrolyzed" and any "hydrolyzed protein," autolyzed yeast, and gelatin.)

- Nitrites and Nitrates

- "Other ingredients"

- Phosphate food additives
- Potassium Bromate
- Propyl Gallate
- Propyl Paraben
- Soy (unless labeled non-GMO and organic)
- Theobromine

When it comes to buying produce, organic and non-genetically modified (non-GMO) is the best option. Localharvest.org lists U.S. farms, co-ops, pick-your-owns, and community supported agriculture (CSAs) for you to find and locally source your food, as well as develop relationships with growers in your area. Traditionally, the Environmental Working Group also provides a list of the dirtiest or most heavily pesticide foods and the cleanest foods.

Creating your meal plan and purchasing food accordingly will help you stay on track by keeping healthy options readily available. Let's not be wasteful, though. Depending on your frequency of shopping, refrigeration, and your climate zone, you may wish to investigate ways to keep your produce fresher longer. Bags, boxes, and refrigerator devices all aim to lengthen the life of your produce. A small investment in this area can prevent throwing your fruits and vegetables in the trash.

REPLENISH:
A well-stocked pantry should contain:

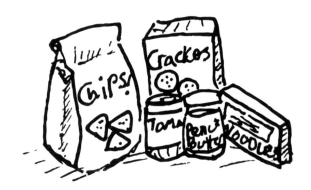

- Coconut oil and extra virgin olive oil
- Glass jars replacing aluminum cans
- Dried fruit
- Dried beans and legumes
- Organic spices
- Organic herbal teas
- Einkorn and organic flours, pasta, and granola

A well-stocked refrigerator should contain:
- Fresh greens
- Seasonal vegetables and fruits
- Raw dairy products
- Almond or coconut milk
- Organic condiments
- Fermented foods

A well-stocked freezer should contain:
- Frozen chicken and beef bone broth
- Frozen organic vegetables and fruits
- 2 to 3 frozen healthy frozen entrees, soups, or stews
- Grass-fed beef, free range chicken, and other protein or wild game
- Pre-homemade breakfast meals (kolaches, einkorn waffles, etc.)

List the common meals you eat at home, the ingredients in them you need to replace, and the healthier ingredients you can use as replacements:

Meal	Ingredients to Replace	Healthier Options
Hot dogs	Nitrates, dyes, corn syrup, margarine, flavorings, preservatives	Kosher all-beef hot dogs without added sodium and nitrates or organic chicken sausage.
Boxed macaroni and cheese	white flour, Maltodextrin, dye, additives	Gluten-free pasta topped with freshly grated raw cheese (optional: add peeled fresh Roma tomato purée and basil leaves).
Can of green beans	BPA, sulfites, sodium	Fresh green beans or organic frozen green beans.
Canned biscuits	Enriched Flour Bleached, Soybean Oil or Hydrogenated oils, Sugar, Aluminum phosphate	Make your own! (recipe at the end of this section)

Einkorn biscuits (alternative to canned biscuits) from the Young Living blog
  2 cups Gary's True Grit™ Einkorn Flour
  1 1/2 tablespoons baking powder
  1 teaspoon salt
  1 tablespoon raw honey
  1/3 cup cold butter
  1/2 cup milk

Instructions:
  1. Preheat oven to 425°F.
  2. In a large bowl, whisk together flour, baking powder, and salt. Add butter and use a pastry cutter to break into small pieces as quickly as possible so butter does not melt. Mixture should resemble coarse meal.
  3. Add honey to milk and mix thoroughly. Gradually stir milk mixture into flour mixture, until dough pulls away from side of bowl.
  4. Place dough on a lightly floured surface and knead 10-15 times. Roll out dough into a 1-inch thick sheet and cut with a cookie cutter or large upside-down glass. Repeat until all dough is used.
  5. Brush off the excess flour and place biscuits onto an ungreased baking sheet.
  6. Bake 13-15 minutes or until edges begin to brown.

> Did you see a trend on your list? Maybe it was a lot of boxed goods or processed foods? Remember that none of these products were available 100 ago and people ate well. No, moms didn't work outside the home, but moms did have to spend a greater deal of time doing things in the home because they also didn't have time-saving devices like dishwashers and electric refrigerators. – Debra Raybern

Please do not let excuses come between you and the life you've always wanted to live. Make a plan to prep meals for the coming weeks. Taking a day or two in a week to pre-cook beans or other proteins will save you time, but still help you put nutritious meals on the table. When age-appropriate, enlist the help of your children, not just as free labor, but as co-chefs in the planning and preparing of meals.

When considering the cost of food, many people believe that healthy food is not worth the expense. However, rather than comparing dollars to dollars, compare calories to calories. Calorie-dense foods such as quinoa, einkorn pasta, basmati rice, and organic beans can be combined with vegetables, meat, and a variety of spices for a healthy meal. If food is prepared for you, it will most likely be more expensive calorie-for-calorie. Fast food and junk food may be cheap, but they are not cost effective.

> The cost of quality ingredients and foods is always cheaper than the cost of disease. – Debra Raybern

Tools for a Healthy Kitchen

Please don't think you must rush out and buy every one of these tools before you can even begin on your journey to wellness because it's not necessary! You can often find tools such as these at garage sales or resale shops. You might even have a friend who's decided to no longer use her kitchen tool. You may ask to borrow it for a while to see if you like it. People may put an item up for sale if they downsized or upgraded to a newer version. Add to your kitchen arsenal of tools over time and as the need arises.

❑ Good set of knives

❑ Juicer – for fresh fruit or vegetable juice with their pulp extracted; pulp may be used in other recipes. Centrifugal are the most common and less expensive; other brands include Breville and JuiceMan. Masticating or cold-press juicers are more expensive, but also extract more nutrients and should leave a dryer pulp than a centrifugal; brands include Omega, Green Star, and Hurom.

❑ Blender – for smoothies, soups, sauces, purees, and juices retaining their fiber. VitaMix and BlendTec are two favorites in this arena, but smaller models for individual servings like the NutriBullet are also effective.

❑ Spiralizer – to turn soft veggies like summer squash and zucchini into pasta-like noodles. There are various manufacturers, so look for features like easy-to-clean and storage to help you decide.

Kids and picky eaters will eat most anything spiraled. – Debra Raybern

❑ Dehydrator – slowly removes the water content of fresh produce or proteins for long term storage. For raw food diets, look for models that have adjustable, low heat options, and a timer like Excalibur.

❑ Slow cooker – to cook meals and meal components slowly without the cook's attention. Slow cookers have been kitchen staple for years; it's like having another cook in the family working through the day or overnight.

❑ Pressure cooker – Today's pressure cooker is electronic, programmable, and doubles as a slow cooker offering the same flavor in less time.

❑ Air fryer – for potato fries, fish, cookies and more. An air fryer is essentially a mini-convection oven. Most require a scant teaspoon or less of oil.

❑ Convection toaster oven – Replace the microwave and avoid heating up the whole house by turning on the oven.

❑ Food processor or slicer/greater/dicer tool – There are endless options, so ask your friends or read consumer reviews for the tool that best meets your need.

Engaging picky eaters in meal planning and grocery shopping often expands their perspective and desire to experiment with food. Sera Johnson, my sister-in-love and the self-proclaimed Former Fast Food Queen, helped her pickiest eater with overcoming new food challenges by having her daughter, Julia, pray before each meal. (You can use this one or create your own.) "Thank you Lord for this good food You made, and thank you for helping me to love Your food." Sera, our co-author of *Nutrition 101: Choose Life!* remembers that, at first, Julia didn't believe her own words, but the more she prayed and spoke those positive words, the more it helped her try new foods and open up her heart to what God provided for her to eat for her health. – Laura Hopkins

My Plan

Copy this sentence in the space below and say it out loud.

"I desire to be well and thrive in life."

_____

My accountability partner(s) is/are:

_____

Track your nutrient intake below or via an app like Lose It and My Fitness Pal.

		Monday	Tuesday	Wednesday	Thursday	Friday	Saturday	Sunday	**Totals**
Protein	Breakfast								
	Lunch								
	Dinner								
Fiber	Breakfast								
	Lunch								
	Dinner								
Sugar	Breakfast								
	Lunch								
	Dinner								
Fat	Breakfast								
	Lunch								
	Dinner								

		Monday	Tuesday	Wednesday	Thursday	Friday	Saturday	Sunday	**Totals**
Protein	Breakfast								
	Lunch								
	Dinner								
Fiber	Breakfast								
	Lunch								
	Dinner								

Sugar	Breakfast								
	Lunch								
	Dinner								
Fat	Breakfast								
	Lunch								
	Dinner								

		Monday	Tuesday	Wednesday	Thursday	Friday	Saturday	Sunday	**Totals**
Protein	Breakfast								
	Lunch								
	Dinner								
Fiber	Breakfast								
	Lunch								
	Dinner								
Sugar	Breakfast								
	Lunch								
	Dinner								
Fat	Breakfast								
	Lunch								
	Dinner								

		Monday	Tuesday	Wednesday	Thursday	Friday	Saturday	Sunday	**Totals**
Protein	Breakfast								
	Lunch								
	Dinner								
Fiber	Breakfast								
	Lunch								
	Dinner								
Sugar	Breakfast								
	Lunch								
	Dinner								

Fat	Breakfast								
	Lunch								
	Dinner								

Now that you have seven days' worth of data charted, let's look at your week.

1. What % was fresh raw fruits and vegetables?

_____

2. What % was fast -food, processed or sugar laden?

_____

3. What % was quality proteins, grains, legumes, dairy, fats or gently cooked veggies.

_____

Now we have picture of a scale with three legs

1. _____%
Optimum: 50%

2. _____%
Optimum: 10% or less

3. _____%
Optimum: 40%

What changes will you make for the remainder of the month?

_____

_____

_____

STEP FOUR
Tune-Up the Body, Mind, and Emotions

STEP FOUR
Tune-Up the Body, Mind, and Emotions

Cleansing

Vehicles and home air conditioning units contain filters, and all car owners and homeowners know that these filters must be checked and changed to keep the machinery and equipment running efficiently and effectively. Your body also contains filters and an elimination system known as your kidneys, liver, and large and small intestines. Cleansing assists the body in removing unwanted toxins and allows the organs to work as they were designed.

For some, cleansing conjures up thoughts of pain and suffering. While there are transitional phases in any cleanse, especially for those new to cleansing, typically those who have positive thoughts up front and are prepared for challenges or cravings will succeed. The benefits of cleansing include increased energy, reduced inflammation, lessened bloating, removal of unwanted toxins, and avoidance of chronic issues.

The question is often posed like this: do I cleanse first, or do I start taking supplements?

One of the very first lessons I learned in herbalist and naturopathic training is to cleanse, then nourish. Cleansing should, for the most part, be gentle yet effective, and something that occurs routinely. No headaches, no rashes, or other major "detox" symptoms should result if the cleanse is done properly and in order; it's vital to listen to the body. However, people with chronic or major health concerns, people on multiple medications, and people who have had a lifetime of toxic exposure and poor eating habits may experience the healing symptoms mentioned on page 24-25. – Debra Raybern

Who should cleanse:
 • Adults
 • Young adults with chronic health issues

Who should not cleanse:
 • Pregnant or nursing mothers – Refer to the section Additional Considerations
 • Children – Lifestyle nutritional changes are preferred for children, but they can benefit from increased fiber and wholesome foods.

When to cleanse?

Quarterly cleansing is ideal for a human body already aligned within a healthy lifestyle. Fewer cleanses for longer periods of time are effective as well. Cleansing should be scheduled and planned in advance to provide the greatest result. The cleanses listed below are meant to be done one at a time, and one each month. Many can be done for as little as a long weekend or one week. This allows the body to rid itself of toxins routinely and not save them up for a massive one-time-per-year dump.

What am I cleansing?

Excess water, toxins, and fats are eliminated through the lungs, the pores of the skin, the kidneys, and the bowels. Removing excess waste from the body and limiting calories will create weight loss, but that should not be the primary reason for cleansing. In fact, if a person returns to his or her unhealthy ways after a cleanse, then it negates the purpose of the cleanse.

How do I prepare?

The best idea is to schedule cleansing for a period of time when you can be at home or in a regular daily routine. Resting physically will allow the body to heal, but often cleansing when going about your daily life makes the day move faster. Preparing meals ahead of time for any family members who are not cleansing is crucial to help you avoid mealtime dilemmas and snacking. Prepare to see worms or parasites eliminated during your cleanse; just remember, it's better for them to leave than to stay inside you.

> When I first started cleansing, I was the only one in my home doing the cleanse, but I still was responsible for feeding everyone else. I highly recommend planning ahead and cooking or preassembling meals that can be frozen or easily put together for those not cleansing. It's not as hard to make meals during a cleanse now that I'm a veteran cleanser, but it was a struggle in the beginning. – Laura Hopkins

Pick a cleanse from the list below and follow it for the time suggested. The "My First Cleanse" week one is a good first choice. Then, as you feel the benefits of your cleanse, you'll be ready to embark on a longer one or to choose a more targeted option from the choices.

If you are new to cleansing or have not done one in over a year, you may want to follow the cleanse that nearly all of my (Debra) clients followed their first month working with me. Instructions on this cleanse is titled "My First Cleanse," and anyone can do it.

Don't try to cleanse every organ all at once; you can always ease into cleansing, especially if this is your first attempt and your diet choices up to now have not been the best. This isn't the 50-yard dash; this is a lifelong marathon. This lifestyle of cleansing and nourishing should be done periodically throughout the rest of your life.

> While going through Master Herbalist school, we were all encouraged to do a cleansing fast for a weekend. Beginning on Friday, we were to eat a healthy lunch, then our next meal wouldn't be until breakfast on Monday morning. I lasted only a few hours; then, I got the shakes, my blood sugar plummeted, I felt light headed, and ran to the refrigerator to eat everything in sight.
>
> I knew from that experience that I needed to make changes that involved more than just adding herbs to my life. I read about many different cleanses and most included fasting along with handfuls of supplements. To say I was not a pill taker is putting it lightly; watching me take a pill was a comedy of horrors, but I'm pleased to say that practice does make perfect and I can now take a pill with ease … one at a time.
>
> As I continued researching, I learned about the Mucousless diet as a cleanse, taught by one of my mentors, Dr. John Christopher. I was free to eat a variety of foods – all that I wanted in fact – according to the plan. I knew I could do it. (Explained on page 59). So, I made sure these foods were in the house, recipes were in hand, and I started my cleanse. To my surprise, I made it with ease to Monday morning. I would later take that successful experience and create a beginner's cleanse for my clients. (page 60) – Debra Raybern

So, give yourself a break. If you have never cleansed before, and by the fifth hour or end of day, you quit – that's ok. Just read through the cleanse options again and pick one that uses real wholesome foods as its base. After a few cleanses are under your belt, you'll be able to tackle any of them with ease. Based on my personal and clinical experience, I recommend several cleanses, all of which are well-suited for beginning cleansers:

1. Debra's 15-Day Clinical Cleanse

2. My First Cleanse

3. A week-long liver cleanse

4. A week-long kidney cleanse

> If you've never cleansed and struggle to stick with it, set yourself up for success by picking a week long cleanse and only do it for just one or two days. Be proud of your accomplishments. Repeat by adding another day. Soon, a week is easy and you'll feel great! Then, you can set up a time to complete the cleanse for the full week. – Debra Raybern

Which cleanse or what products do I use?
There are many cleansing kits on the market, and many accomplish specific tasks. So, the goals of the cleanser should be considered. It is generally accepted that the colon must be eliminating well first so the toxins collected can be freely eliminated, which will often prevent the unwanted side effects some people experience with a cleanse.

What about food on the cleanse?
All of the cleanses listed below utilize fresh food. Changing your current eating to all healthy and 50% raw foods is a cleanse in itself.

> You may try to ease into a cleanse mentally by substituting one meal a day with a shake or smoothies made with Balance Complete™, Power Meal, or Pure Protein Complete™ powders and raw fruits or vegetables. – Laura Hopkins

What about colonics and coffee enemas?
Colonics and coffee enemas are almost always mentioned in regards to any type of cleansing. Either option significantly speeds up the cleansing process, especially in connection with the liver.

Colonic
A colonic is the infusion of water into the rectum by a colon therapist to cleanse and flush out the colon. It is also called colonic hydrotherapy or colon irrigation.

Consult with local chiropractors, massage therapists and health food stores to find a colon hydrotherapist in your area. Search "at home colonic equipment" to find the tools for a self-administered colonic if a therapist is not in your area.

Coffee enema
The ancient Egyptians used rectal cleansing; however, coffee was not used until 1917, and this method appeared in the Merck Manual until 1972. German researchers studied caffeine's effect on the bile duct and small intestines in the 1920s. Founder of the Gerson Institute, Max Gerson proposed that coffee enemas were unlike saline enemas because the caffeine traveled through the smooth muscle of the small intestine and into the liver, clearing even more of the gastro-intestinal tract and removing more toxins and bile than a normal saline enema. He believed coffee enemas were most beneficial for the function and the stimulation of the liver. There is plenty of research online and books at your local library or on Amazon, and there are coffee enema kits available for purchase too.

Effective Cleansing Options

Cleansing Trio™ (Young Living Essential Oils product)
Ideal for anyone new to cleansing or for those with ongoing digestive challenges. The three supplements – Essentialzyme™, ICP™, and ComforTone® – in this cleanse can be used with a healthy diet for 30 days. Augmented with herbs that are rich in vitamins, minerals, enzymes, amino acids, fiber, and essential oils, the Cleansing Trio™ is designed specifically to cleanse the colon.

Daniel Fast – One to 30 days
Based on the Biblical account of the prophet Daniel, this cleansing diet can be used for extended periods of time. It allows consumption of all fruit, vegetables, whole grains, nuts and seeds, legumes, and quality oils. Acceptable beverages include water, unsweetened almond milk, coconut milk, rice milk, or soy milk, as well as herbs, spices, salt, pepper, unsweetened coconut flakes, seasonings, Bragg's Liquid Amino's, soy products, and tofu. To avoid soy, select coconut-based amino acids.

Five-Day Nutritive Cleanse (Young Living Essential Oils product)
Many have found success with this program that incorporates Balance Complete™ as a meal replacement shake, NingXia Red®, Digest + Cleanse™ capsules, and healthy quantities of pure, clean water. Instructions come with the program components.

Juicing Cleanses – One meal to 30 days
An all-liquid juicing cleanse can be very effective, but requires extensive planning and specific equipment. Just as with any cleanse, it's best to slowly ease into a cooked diet upon completion by increasing water intake, cutting out caffeine, and eating more raw fruits and vegetables. All juice cleanses should begin with warm water with lemon first thing in the morning to stimulate the liver, and it's a good habit to continue after a scheduled cleanse to promote continued health. Be diligent about drinking juices every 2 to 3 hours, even when you are not hungry because consistency is healing and skipping a juice could tank your blood sugar, creating additional issues. In many juice cleanse programs, if you find yourself very hungry, you may eat the raw version of the food you are juicing for the added fiber to feel full.

Master Cleanse
Stanley Burroughs developed this process in the 1950s, and there have been many variations of it over the years. Also called the Lemonade Diet, it is intended to provide a healthy number of calories and nutrients specifically suited for cleansing, all while resting the digestive system and allowing the body to heal naturally. The concept is that the ingredients, all easily acquired at local health food stores or online, promote the body to move from an acidic pH to an alkaline pH. Generally, this cleanse lasts from 10 to 21 days, but extended cleansing can be done for chronic issues. This is the cleanse many people had problems with when it was their first attempt at a cleanse, and their diet beforehand was the Standard American Diet (SAD) of processed, refined, sugary foods. After a few other cleanses and dietary improvements, the Master Cleanse was then enjoyed.

> A few clients follow this cleanse for three to five days, then entered the 15-Day Cleanse as their first entree into cleansing. – Debra Raybern

Three-Day Detox and Mucusless
Preparation of the body through a three-day detox makes way for the strategic mucusless diet and a more alkaline body. It includes prune and apple juices, clean water, and tablespoons of olive oil to act as a lubricator for the first three days, and then whole, live, and raw foods. Essentially this is a vegan diet with lots of juicing.

Saunas – A great addition to other cleanses or as your chosen cleanse.

Sweating is a great way to release toxins through your skin during the cleanse. The heat of the sauna increases the core body temperature, causing blood vessels to dilate and blood flow to increase. The heat moves toward the surface of the skin where millions of sweat glands respond to signals from the nervous system to start producing sweat to cool the body. Deep sweating in the sauna can help reduce toxins in the body absorbed just from our daily environment. Types of saunas include dry, steam, and far-infrared, and information for each may be found through basic research. Many gyms, fitness centers, and even some health food stores offer saunas.

My First Cleanse

Eating all vegan foods, meaning no animal products including dairy and eggs, for one week, with 50% of the food in its raw, un-cooked state. You may consume all of the fresh fruit and vegetables you want, provided they are in their raw state. So, no heating or processing is allowed. These foods may be consumed via juices, blender drinks, salads or eating them directly from the refrigerator. You are not limited to the amount of foods to consume. You will want to be sure you consume enough that you don't become so hungry that you go back to eating the normal way. The following program has been successful for many:

- First thing in the morning, drink eight ounces of warm water with the juice of one lemon.

- Thirty minutes later, drink eight ounces of a fresh fruit drink.

- Midmorning eat approximately 10 soaked almonds* and another eight ounces of fresh fruit or vegetable juice.

- Lunch consists of a nice tossed salad with a variety of shredded vegetables and nutritious seeds or nuts, such as sunflower, pumpkin, or Chia.

- A mid-afternoon snack consists of a fresh nut butter on raw seed crackers or carrot sticks or celery. Another eight ounces of fresh vegetable juice including carrot, beet, and greens such as spinach or kale.

- Dinner consists of another large salad with steamed vegetables and your choice of protein, fish, or grilled chicken. If you prefer to stay completely vegan, you may add legumes too.

Debra's 15-Day Clinical Cleanse

Combining highly effective components of three different cleanses, you begin with a meal replacement shake (Balance Complete™), colon cleansing powder (ICP™), and enzymes (EssentialZymes 4+™). If needed to have the bowels move two to three times per day, add ComforTone® capsules to stimulate peristalsis or movement of the colon. This is a great cleanse to start off the year with, after those months of extra eating and enjoyment of holiday foods.

Days 1-5: Breakfast lunch and dinner consists of a Balance Complete™ Shake made according to directions. This shake contains superfood nutrients and 11 grams of Young Living's proprietary V-Fiber blend, which helps with the feeling of fullness. You may make it with water and ice, or rice, coconut, or almond milk. Take the cleansing powder and enzymes as directed on the bottle. Drink plenty of water in between meals and smell peppermint oil if you start to get hungry.

Days 6-10: Follow My First Cleanse above.

Days 11-15: Follow the Master Cleanse on page 59.

Day 16+: Ease back into eating with fresh raw fruits and vegetables during the day; for dinner enjoy a baked potato with the skin on or with a drizzle of olive oil and salt-free seasoning. Remember your goal is to NOT return to your old eating habits. So, during these 15 days, you will be learning and selecting the diet plan that you will begin after this cleanse.

Two Additional Clinical Cleanses

Designed specifically for the liver and kidneys, these should be done separately, preferably during a month where a different cleanse is not chosen, or you just are giving your liver and kidneys some extra love.

5-Day Liver Cleanse

Follow this routine for five consecutive days, but do not do the liver/gallbladder drink at the same time as the kidney cleanse drink as listed below in the Kidney Cleanse. Space each cleanse at least one week apart.
- Upon rising, drink eight ounces of distilled water.
- Prepare the Liver Flush drink as outlined below and drink.
- After one hour, drink your morning green drink: 1 Tbsp. JuvaPower® (YLEO) with eight ounces fresh fruit juice in water.
- Until noon, consume only fresh fruit juices, liquefied ripe fruit drinks, smoothies, and water.
- For lunch you can have raw vegetable juices, raw vegetable salads or potassium broth (see below).
- Afternoon snacks can be raw vegetables, herbal teas, potassium broth, or sprouts.
- Dinner can be diluted fruit juices and smoothies, fresh fruit salads, and herbal teas.
- Consume at least five cloves of raw garlic every day. Yes, during this five-day cleanse you will smell like garlic. Use your Thieves® toothpaste and mouthwash or add a drop of cinnamon essential oil to Slique™ Gum to freshen your breath.
- Be sure to consume three to four quarts of distilled water daily. No eggs, dairy, meat, salt, sugar, tofu, breads, pasta, coffee, sodas, or processed foods. NO cooked foods for the entire five days. When you do return to eating cooked foods on day six, start with steamed vegetables or a baked potato with olive oil and spices. Do not add butter, so as not to jolt your system.

Liver & Gallbladder Flush Drink

In a blender mix the following:
- 8 ounces of fresh orange or other citrus juice, apple juice or grape juice. (Debra likes grapefruit, and Laura prefers orange)
- 1-5 cloves of garlic (Start with one clove on Day 1 and increase by one clove each day.)
- 1-5 tablespoons first, cold-pressed olive oil (Start with one Tbsp. on Day 1 and increase by one Tbsp. each day.)
- 1 one-inch piece ginger, peeled

5-Day Kidney Cleanse

Follow this routine for five consecutive days, but do not do the Kidney Cleanse at the same time as the Liver/Gallbladder cleanse. Space each cleanse at least one week apart.
- Upon rising, drink eight ounces of distilled water.
- Prepare the Kidney Flush drink as outlined below and drink.
- After one hour, drink your morning green drink: 1 Tbsp. JuvaPower® (YLEO) with eight ounces fresh fruit juice in water.
- Until noon, consume only fresh fruit juices, liquefied ripe fruit drinks, smoothies, and water.
- For lunch, you can have raw vegetable juices, raw vegetable salads or potassium broth (see below).
- Afternoon snacks can be raw vegetables, herbal teas, potassium broth, or sprouts.
- Dinner can be diluted fruit juices and smoothies, fresh fruit salads, and herbal teas.
- Consume at least five cloves of raw garlic every day. Yes, during this five-day cleanse you will smell like garlic. Use your Thieves® toothpaste and mouthwash or add a drop of cinnamon essential oil to Slique™ Gum to freshen your breath.

• Be sure to consume three to four quarts of distilled water daily. No eggs, dairy, meat, salt, sugar, tofu, breads, pasta, coffee, sodas, or processed foods. NO cooked foods for the entire five days. When you do return to eating cooked foods on day six, start with steamed vegetables or a baked potato with olive oil and spices. Do not add butter, so as not to jolt your system.

Kidney Flush Drink
In a blender, mix the following:
   • Juice of one lemon or lime. If organic, put half a lemon into the blender and let it pulverize.
   • 16 ounces of distilled water
   • A pinch of cayenne powder
   • Small amount of maple syrup or Yacon for flavoring

*Potassium Broth Recipe
Use only organically grown vegetables.
   • Fill a large soup pot with 25% potato peelings, 25% carrot peelings and whole chopped beets, 25% chopped onions, 25% celery and dark greens, and 50 (fifty) cloves of garlic.
   • Add a few hot peppers and fill the pot with enough distilled water to cover the vegetables.
   • Simmer on low temperature for two hours or more.
   • Strain and reserve the broth. Vegetables can go to the compost heap.
   • Drink the broth freely throughout the day.

Additional Recipes

For juices made in a juicer not a blender, pour any leftovers into a glass jar. Store it in the refrigerator and enjoy within 24 hours.

Green Juice
 1 Green apple, sliced to fit into the juicer
 1 carrot
 1 leaf kale, no stalk
 1/4 lemon wedge

Juice all ingredients and pour over ice.

Green Apple Lemonade
Kids and adults love this lemonade. Makes a great afternoon drink.

 6 green apples
 1 small to medium lemon sliced to fit into the juicer

Juice all ingredients and pour over ice.

Morning Start Juice
 1 small peeled grapefruit, sliced to fit into the juicer
 1/2 red apple
 1/3 medium pineapple, peeled unless your juicer can handle the outside, sliced to fit into the juicer

Green Smoothie
 2 Tbsp. flaxseed
 2 Tbsp. Chia seeds
 2 Tbsp. sesame seeds
 1 cup cold, clean water
 1/2 cup ice
 1 medium peeled orange
 1/2 avocado
 1 cup spinach
 1 cup or 2-3 kale leaves
 1 scoop of Pure Protein Complete™ (optional)

In a blender combine the flaxseeds, sesame seeds, and Chia seeds; blend until it has the consistency of flour. Turn off the blender and scrape the sides of the blender to loosen the seed flour. Add the rest of the ingredients and blend until creamy. Add more water or fresh juice as desired.

Red Velvet Juice

This name is a nod to texture and color, not flavor. Be mindful that beets are powerful detoxifiers and consuming large quantities is not recommended. Beets, also known as beetroot, last longer in the refrigerator if you cut off the beet top because the root still supplies moisture to the leaves. The beet top can be eaten too and is delicious sautéed.

    1 whole organic lemon
    1 one small or half of a medium-sized organic beet without the beet top (leaves).

Drink the juice and add the pulp to the compost.

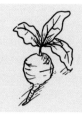

Clients who consumed beets in salads or in juice would call my office in a panic. A peek at the morning toilet bowel had them seeing red, but there was (and is) no reason to worry. Red stools reveal the beet's deep color coming out and eliminating naturally. – Debra Raybern

Morning Buzz

    1 heaping teaspoon of AlkaLime®
    8 ounces of distilled water
    1 tube NingXia Nitro®

Combine all in a glass (leave plenty of room for the AlkaLime® to rise, stir, and enjoy immediately.

Mint Chocolate Morning

    2 scoops of Chocolate Pure Protein Complete™
    2 drops Peppermint Vitality™ oil
    1 teaspoon Chia seeds

Mix and enjoy. The Chia seeds will become gelatinous, a texture that kids often enjoy.

Audrey's Concoction

    1 scoop Balance Complete™
    1 scoop Vanilla Pure Protein Complete™
    1 cup frozen papaya, mango, and pineapple
    8 ounces of water

Blend the water and frozen fruit first and then add the powders for a smoother shake. Add more water if you want a thinner consistency.

The Mind

The field of Epigenetics is teaching us a lot of truth about how our genetic codes are not a definite possibility. We have the ability to alter DNA from generation to generation with lifestyle choices and even a changed perspective on life through healthy thought patterns. Renewing the mind can bring powerful and long-lasting effects, but it is a daily, step-by-step process.

Have you heard …
   "Your beliefs become your thoughts,
   Your thoughts become your words,
   Your words become your actions,
   Your actions become your habits,
   Your habits become your values, and
   Your values become your destiny."

Belief is *essential* to your wellness. If you do not think you deserve to be well, or that you can be, chances are that you will not embrace your *Road to Wellness*.

So, it's time to take inventory of what you believe and think about your health. Do you believe that you can be healthy? Is there a broken link in this chain reaction of who you are and who you desire to become? What thoughts do you desire to give up, and what thoughts do you desire to magnify?

Wrong belief or thought patterns:

_____

_____

_____

_____

Our minds need a detox as well! Pull the plug on those
feelings that aren't serving you! – Debra Raybern

Realigned, destiny-fulling thought patterns about my health, body image, genetics:

_____

_____

_____

_____

Emotions

We all have, should, and will continue to experience emotions, both positive and negative ones, on a daily basis. It's part of the human experience. At times, these emotions may add stress which then affects the body in a physical way. The key is being in charge of the emotions, fully accepting or rejecting them, and releasing those that do not serve you in a positive or progressive way. Mastering the thought life will aid you tremendously in mastering your emotions and vice versa. Because the body is also part of this triad, the negative emotions that you choose to hold onto or that are trapped most definitely impact your physical health for the long term.

Negative emotions I desire to release:

_____

_____

_____

_____

Positive emotions I am ready to restore or magnify:

_____

_____

_____

_____

This is not a one-time negative-emotion removal. Because you are a human and interact with other humans, you will continue to need emotional releases. You can also choose to use the following supplements from Young Living that provide support for the endocrine system and emotions.

- ❏ Estro™
- ❏ FemiGen™
- ❏ Mineral Essence™
- ❏ PD 80/20™
- ❏ Prenolone® Plus Body Cream
- ❏ EndoGize™
- ❏ Prostate Health™
- ❏ CortiStop®
- ❏ Thyromin™

When you experience negative emotions, you have the choice to hold onto the emotion or let it go. We like to apply essential oils to our head and heart and say, "I lovingly and willingly release these emotions that do not serve me in a positive or progressive way." Imagine yourself taking that emotion or burden physically off your body as you would a weed, pulling all of the roots from the ground, and separating it from yourself. Then, begin to apply oils and speak positive words to fill up the area of your emotions that was cleared. – Laura Hopkins

The following chart shows a number of blends that help with the release of emotions. Think of these oils as tools. When you decide to diffuse or wear the blend Harmony™, pause and consider if you have any relationships that are less than harmonious; now decide how you will repair this issue and restore harmony. Do you need passion in your life? Then, wear some Live Your Passion™ oil blend and say to yourself throughout the day, "I live each moment passionately as if it were my last." At the end of the week you may find your cup overflowing with passion for life.

Oils for the Emotions

Oil	Emotion	Worn/Diffused	Words of Affirmation
Believe™	Lack of self confidence	Wrists and smell	I am a strong and confident person.

Essential Oils for Feelings and Emotional Support from Young Living:

- ❑ Acceptance™
- ❑ Awaken™
- ❑ Believe™
- ❑ Clarity™
- ❑ Common Sense™
- ❑ Dream Catcher™
- ❑ Envision™
- ❑ Forgiveness™
- ❑ Gathering™
- ❑ Gratitude™
- ❑ Grounding™
- ❑ Harmony™
- ❑ Highest Potential™
- ❑ Hope™
- ❑ Humility™
- ❑ Inner Child™
- ❑ Inspiration™
- ❑ Into the Future™
- ❑ Joy™
- ❑ Live Your Passion™
- ❑ Magnify Your Purpose™
- ❑ Motivation™
- ❑ Oola® Balance™
- ❑ Oola® Grow™
- ❑ Peace & Calming® or Peace & Calming II™
- ❑ Present Time™
- ❑ Release™
- ❑ Sacred Mountain™
- ❑ SARA™
- ❑ Stress Away™
- ❑ Surrender™
- ❑ 3 Wise Men™
- ❑ Trauma Life™
- ❑ Tranquil™
- ❑ Transformation™
- ❑ Valor® or Valor II™
- ❑ White Angelica™

My Plan

Copy this sentence in the space below and say it out loud.
"I desire to be well and thrive in life."

_____

I choose to cleanse _____ times a year using the _____

_____

The dates I will cleanse are _____

_____

I lovingly and willingly choose to release the trapped emotion of _____
that does not serve me in a positive or progressive way.

I lovingly and willingly choose to release the trapped emotion of _____
that does not serve me in a positive or progressive way.

I lovingly and willingly choose to release the trapped emotion of _____
that does not serve me in a positive or progressive way.

Positive emotions I choose to restore or magnify: _____

_____

_____

_____

Realigned, destiny-fulling thought patterns about my health, body image, genetics: _____

_____

_____

_____

My accountability partner(s) is/are

_____

STEP FIVE
Nourish and Replenish

STEP FIVE
Nourish and Replenish

It takes the body about 90 days for cells to rejuvenate or replenish and for you to establish good habits. So, let's review your first 90 days to be sure you're on track for success.

Let's recap what you've done thus far:

Month 1:
- ❑ Obtain your baseline blood work through various testing and record the results on page 22.
- ❑ Complete the Goals Chart on page 24 so you know where you are headed.
- ❑ Successfully revamp the whole house to replace all chemically-laden products and foods with healthy alternatives.
- ❑ Choose one or a combination of eating plans to begin.

Month 2:
- ❑ Pick a cleanse and follow for at least one week.
- ❑ Continue with your new and healthy eating plan.
- ❑ Begin "My First Plan" or one of the five-day cleanses for the liver or kidney.
- ❑ Spend time thinking about and journaling the thoughts and emotions that may be hindering you from living the life you desire
- ❑ Take necessary steps to remove these hindrances.
- ❑ Add specific supplements and essential oils that support your journey to wellness.

Month 3:
- ❑ Set aside five days this month to do another five-day cleanse or other cleanse of your choice. Remember all of the cleanses work on the whole body. The Cleansing Trio™ concentrates on the digestive system, and of course the 5-Day Liver cleanse focuses on the liver and the 5-Day Kidney on the kidneys. The others are whole body cleanses. By the end of 12 months, we hope you will have used all of the cleanses at least once. Even if this is just your second cleanse, you will have obtained great improvements by now.
- ❑ Now it's time to create your own "Homework for Health" plan for your next 90 days.
- ❑ If you have not already, begin to Nourish with NingXia Red®, OmegaGize3™, and MultiGreens™. The supplements are taken as directed on the bottle.
- ❑ Select and use essential oils.

Your actions will follow your beliefs. Now that your first 90 days has you feeling refreshed, energized, and empowered to take control of your own wellness and eager to do even more, where should you head next? Do you have another three months to achieve greater vitality? Three more months to get rid of annoying health challenges? YES, YOU DO! It's your health, and you are committed to your own wellness!

Only you can take responsibility and make the commitment to be successful and live the energetic, vitality-filled life of wellness you desire. Now that you have made significant changes, this next three month plan we call Homework for Health, allows you to create a custom plan so you can achieve the desired results. Over 80% of clients who followed this plan, never needed to have a coaching session with me (Debra) because their health challenges were resolved or were resolving, and they gained valuable empowerment to use good nutrition, the Young Living products, great nutrition and lifestyle changes to create wellness for themselves.

You stocked your refrigerator and pantry, but how about your library? Knowledge isn't just power for your mind, it's power to your health. Nutrition is a must. It must be wholesome – not fast food or full of preservatives. By now, you get that! Now is the right time to purchase *Nutrition 101: Choose Life!* It's the premier nutrition primer for all ages and an excellent recipe and resource guide to help you move from unhealthy eating habits to creating a culture of healthy choices. Simply put, it is a life changer. Order online at www.growinghealthyhomes.com.

Nutrition 101: Choose Life! was required reading and implements for all my clients. – Debra Raybern

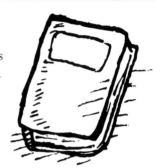

Are you using the Young Living products? Then THE book to learn about the products and suggestions for specific challenges is the *Essential Oil Desk Reference* or *Essential Oil Pocket Reference*. If you do not own one, it is a must have for using the oils to their maximum benefit, for restoring your health, and taking care of your family. Learn about each oil, supplement, and alternatives to toxic filled commercial products. It will aid you tremendously as you maintain your journey on the Road to Wellness. The desk version contains a wealth of knowledge to be gained. Purchase it from the publisher at www.discoverlsp.com.

Now it's time to create your next 90-day plan. The following example is easy to follow, but still you may modify it for your personal needs and to keep you feeling your best.

Supplements:
- ❑ NingXia Red® – one ounce per day. Option to add one to three drops each of the following YLEO Vitality™ dietary line of oils designed to be taken orally: DiGize™, Carrot Seed, and Frankincense.
- ❑ Core Supplements™ pack – Master Formula™, Life 9™, Longevity™ softgels, and OmegaGize³™ packaged in a daily sachet and taken as directed on the box.
- ❑ Essentialzyme™ or Essentialzymes-4™ or Detoxzyme® (vegan formula) taken as directed on bottle or box. Pick one, not all.
- ❑ Slique™ Tea – one cup per day if weight balance is the challenge

Essential Oils:
- ❑ The Feelings™ Kit – Select one oil from this kit or the list of mind/emotional oil blends on page 68 and wear them on your wrists or over your heart each day. Also smell the same oil twice per day for at least one minute per oil. Alternate oils so you concentrate on a different oil from the kit daily. As you smell each oil, look at the name on the bottle and reflect on this emotion and how it may apply to you. Emotions have a profound impact on the physical body. Stress accounts for 80% of all diseases according to the American Medical Association and National Institute of Health. We must take control of all the stressors in life, both physical and emotional.
- ❑ ImmuPower™ blend – Wear one drop on your chest in the morning and one drop on the bottom of each foot at bedtime to support the immune system.
- ❑ Valor® or Valor II™ – Place one drop on the bottom of each foot at bedtime.
- ❑ Peace & Calming® or Peace & Calming II™ – Place one drop on the bottom of each foot at bedtime.

All oils applied to the feet may be layered one after the other, or the drops in the palm of the hand, stirred clockwise and then applied as a combination.
- ❑ Purification® – Diffuse five drops daily
- ❑ Lemon – Diffuse five drops daily
- ❑ Thieves® – Diffuse two drops daily
- ❑ Joy™ – Diffuse two drops daily

All of these oils may be combined and diffused together; if combined, one drop each works well. Diffuse them in a room where you will be for 30 minutes daily.

Other must do's:

Exercise at least 20 minutes per day. Be sure the type of exercise selected fits in with your ability and current health status. Consult a medical doctor or personal trainer if unsure.

Stop using chemical cleaners and chemically-laden body care and bath products. Switch to the many products offered by Young Living. Stop any and all use of bleach products; the Thieves® Household Cleaner will clean and disinfect.

Stop the use of the microwave. Unplug it, or completely remove it from the kitchen.

No substitution of supplements or oils with those of another company. This is important! We picked Young Living because they work!

Select three other supplements or oils for the top three symptoms you are experiencing and write them below:

_____

_____

_____

I used other essential oils, but it was only the Young Living brand that
produced the results I desired for clients. – Debra Raybern

Here are some recommended supplements listed by body system. Learn about each in the Product Guide, product information sheets in the Young Living Virtual Office, or in one of the reference books.

Brain and Nervous System
- ❏ Master Formula™
- ❏ Mineral Essence™
- ❏ MultiGreens™
- ❏ NingXia Nitro®
- ❏ NingXia Red®
- ❏ NingXia Wolfberries
- ❏ OmegaGize³™

Digestive System
- ❏ AlkaLime®
- ❏ Allerzyme™
- ❏ ComforTone®
- ❏ Detoxzyme®
- ❏ Digest + Cleanse™
- ❏ Essentialzyme™
- ❏ Essentialzymes-4™
- ❏ ICP™
- ❏ Inner Defense™
- ❏ JuvaPower®
- ❏ JuvaSpice®
- ❏ JuvaTone®
- ❏ Life 9™
- ❏ ParaFree™
- ❏ Rehemogen™

Respiratory System
- ❏ Inner Defense™
- ❏ Life 9™
- ❏ NingXia Red®
- ❏ Super C™

Auditory System
- ❏ Detoxzyme®
- ❏ Inner Defense™
- ❏ NingXia Red®
- ❏ Sulfurzyme®
- ❏ Super C™

Visual
- ❏ Longevity™ Softgels
- ❏ Master Formula™
- ❏ Mineral Essence™
- ❏ MultiGreens™
- ❏ NingXia Red®
- ❏ OmegaGize³™

Skeletal/Muscular System
- ❏ AlkaLime®
- ❏ AgiLease™
- ❏ Essentialzyme™
- ❏ Essentialzymes-4™
- ❏ Master Formula™
- ❏ MegaCal™

Cardiovascular System
- ❏ AlkaLime®
- ❏ Longevity™ Softgels
- ❏ Master Formula™
- ❏ MegaCal™
- ❏ Mineral Essence™
- ❏ MultiGreens™
- ❏ NingXia Nitro®
- ❏ NingXia Red®
- ❏ NingXia Wolfberries
- ❏ OmegaGize³™
- ❏ Rehemogen™
- ❏ Super B™
- ❏ Super Cal™

Immune System
- ❏ Digest + Cleanse™
- ❏ ImmuPro™
- ❏ Inner Defense™
- ❏ Life 5™
- ❏ Master Formula™
- ❏ Mineral Essence™
- ❏ MultiGreens™
- ❏ NingXia Nitro®
- ❏ NingXia Red®
- ❏ NingXia Wolfberries
- ❏ OmegaGize³™
- ❏ ParaFree™
- ❏ Sulfurzyme®
- ❏ Super C™

Endocrine System
- ❏ CortiStop®
- ❏ EndoGize™
- ❏ Estro™
- ❏ FemiGen™
- ❏ Master Formula™
- ❏ Mineral Essence™
- ❏ NingXia Nitro®
- ❏ NingXia Red®
- ❏ OmegaGize³™
- ❏ PD 80/20™
- ❏ Prenolone® Plus Body Cream
- ❏ Progessence Plus™
- ❏ Prostate Health™
- ❏ Protec™
- ❏ Thyromin™

My Plan

Copy this sentence in the space below and say it out loud.

"I desire to be well and thrive in life."

_____

Return to the chart in STEP THREE on page 21 that listed your test results. Record the supplements you will use in the sixth column.

I have the following supplements:_____

_____

_____

to support the following systems: _____

_____

_____

I will purchase the following supplements:_____

_____

_____

to support the following systems: _____

_____

_____

My accountability partner(s) is/are:

_____

STEP SIX
Oiling Up

STEP SIX
Oiling Up

Most people who begin with Young Living Essential Oils start with oils, but we've chosen to include them at the end of this process. Why? Having a great foundation for health through the previous steps will make your use of essential oils much more effective. Oils have specific assignments in creation, but all of the junk we allow into our environment and bodies can slow down the long-term impact of essential oils.

If you're working through this manual with a different brand of essential oils or supplements, we would like to caution you. The authors only endorse the use of YL products based on a combined 27 years of experience using them. We only recommend Young Living because we are confident in the quality of the products because of the Seed to Seal® guarantee of this 23+ year-old company.

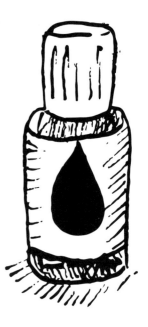

Applications

There are many, many books on the proper application techniques and purposes for the oils. The following is the most basic information and guidelines for application. It's always best to think about what result you want to experience from an oil to determine which application method to use. Consult a reference book for best results.

Inhale/Diffuse

Direct inhalation of an oil takes it through the nasal passages, up to the olfactory system, and into the limbic system. This central brain is responsible for memory and is considered the feeling portion of the brain. Your sense of smell is wired directly to it while your other four senses (sight, sound, taste, and touch) are wired to the frontal lobe or the reasoning brain. To inhale, smell oils from the bottle, a cotton ball, or from a drop placed in the palm of your hand.

Diffusing is a simple and effective way to impact your environment. In fact, it's so powerful that the small molecular structure of diffused essential oils allows it to pass through sheetrock in a building from room to room, even where there is no hallway or door connecting the rooms.[1] These molecules also linger, clinging to every surface they can penetrate, just like the residue of cigarette smoking does.

After I (Laura) moved from one home to another, the new owner and my friend did some remodeling. When I returned to admire the work, two other friends were there and all commented that it still "smelled" like my house. Eight years of diffusing essential oils still permeated the atmosphere. Likewise, those oils are permeating the porous surface of our bodies and also traveling via the same method of inhalation.

Topical

The skin is your largest organ and absorbs essential oils easily; whatever you absorb externally has an internal impact on the internal environment. You may apply the oils neat (undiluted) to the skin or undiluted.

If an oil feels uncomfortably warm or seems to irritate the skin, just apply a good quality carrier oil, like V-6™ Complex, and that will dilute the oil at the surface of the skin, allowing for a slower rate of descent into the body. Irritation is often not due to the oil, but because the previous exposure of the skin to petrochemicals and toxins, which causes the oils to react. If you are unsure about where to apply an oil or concerned about potential irritation, you can always apply the oils neat (undiluted) to the feet.

Raindrop Technique is a non-invasive method of anointing the feet and back with oils in a systematic way that allows for relaxation and detoxification. Although anyone can learn to perform a Raindrop, make sure you receive and are taught by someone with knowledge of the oils, who only uses Young Living, and aligns with your belief system. Drink plenty of water before and after, as you would a massage, to help flush any toxins that the oils evict from your body.

Internal

We wholeheartedly support the ingestion of Young Living essential oils. The Vitality™ line of oils is specifically labeled for use as a dietary supplement. You may choose to add oils to water or liquids to drink, in empty vegetable capsules, or to food. The quickest way to get oils into the bloodstream is to put a drop directly under the tongue and onto the soft tissues of the mouth.

[1] Nature's RX

Organized by body system, the following oils are our top (not exhaustive) list of essential oils to use:

Vitality™ oils for ingestion or cooking

- ❏ Basil
- ❏ Bergamot
- ❏ Black Pepper
- ❏ Cardamom
- ❏ Carrot Seed
- ❏ Celery Seed
- ❏ Cinnamon Bark
- ❏ Citrus Fresh
- ❏ Clove
- ❏ Copaiba
- ❏ Coriander
- ❏ DiGize™
- ❏ Dill
- ❏ EndoFlex™
- ❏ Fennel
- ❏ Frankincense
- ❏ GLF™
- ❏ German Chamomile
- ❏ Ginger
- ❏ Grapefruit
- ❏ Jade Lemon™
- ❏ JuvaCleanse®
- ❏ JuvaFlex®
- ❏ Laurus Nobilis
- ❏ Lavender
- ❏ Lemon
- ❏ Lemongrass
- ❏ Lime
- ❏ Longevity™
- ❏ Marjoram
- ❏ Mountain Savory
- ❏ Nutmeg
- ❏ Orange
- ❏ Oregano
- ❏ Peppermint
- ❏ Rosemary
- ❏ Sage
- ❏ SclarEssence™
- ❏ Spearmint
- ❏ Tangerine
- ❏ Tarragon
- ❏ Thieves®
- ❏ Thyme

Brain

- ❏ Frankincense
- ❏ Sacred Frankincense
- ❏ Vetiver
- ❏ Brain Power™

Digestive System

- ❏ Peppermint
- ❏ Spearmint
- ❏ AromaEase™
- ❏ DiGize™
- ❏ JuvaCleanse®
- ❏ JuvaFlex®

Respiratory System

- ❏ Breathe Again™
- ❏ Eucalyptus Blue/Globulus
- ❏ Laurus Nobilis
- ❏ Myrtle
- ❏ Eucalyptus Radiata
- ❏ R.C.™

Olfactory System

- ❏ Basil

Auditory System

- ❏ Helichrysum
- ❏ Awaken™
- ❏ Melrose™

Visual

- ❏ Cypress
- ❏ Frankincense
- ❏ Sacred Frankincense

Muscular/Skeletal System
- ❏ Basil
- ❏ Copaiba
- ❏ Idaho Blue Spruce
- ❏ Lemongrass
- ❏ Marjoram
- ❏ Tea Tree
- ❏ Oregano
- ❏ Peppermint
- ❏ Thyme
- ❏ Wintergreen
- ❏ Aroma Siez™
- ❏ Deep Relief™
- ❏ PanAway®
- ❏ Relieve It™
- ❏ Thieves®
- ❏ Xiang Mao (Red lemongrass)
- ❏ Valor® or Valor II™

Cardiovascular System
- ❏ Amazonian Ylang Ylang
- ❏ Helichrysum
- ❏ Marjoram
- ❏ Aroma Life™

Immune System
- ❏ Laurus Nobilis
- ❏ Oregano
- ❏ Sacred Frankincense
- ❏ Xiang Mao (Red lemongrass)
- ❏ Thieves®

Endocrine system
- ❏ Amazonian Ylang Ylang
- ❏ Clary Sage
- ❏ Coriander
- ❏ Fennel
- ❏ Goldenrod
- ❏ Hinoki
- ❏ Idaho Balsam Fir
- ❏ Jasmine
- ❏ Myrrh
- ❏ EndoFlex™
- ❏ ScarlEssence™
- ❏ Shutran™
- ❏ Dragon Time™
- ❏ Lady Sclareol™
- ❏ Sensation™

My Plan

Copy this sentence in the space below and say it out loud.

"I desire to be well and thrive in life."

_____

Return to the chart in STEP THREE on page 21 that listed your test results. Record the essential oils you will use in the sixth column.

I will commit to finding someone who can perform the Raindrop Technique on me at least _____ times a quarter and _____ times a year.

I have the following essential oils: _____

_____

_____

to support the following systems: _____

_____

_____

I will purchase the following essential oils: _____

_____

_____

to support the following systems: _____

_____

_____

My accountability partner(s) is/are:

_____

STEP SEVEN
Journey On

STEP SEVEN
Journey On

We are coming to the end of *Road to Wellness*, but your journey has just started! You are equipped with the tools to make healthy, successful choices and live the energetic, vitality filled life of wellness you desire.

> More than 80% of people who follow this plan never needed to have a coaching session with me as their health challenges were resolved or were resolving, and they gained valuable empowerment that they can use the Young Living products, great nutrition, and lifestyle changes to create wellness themselves. In fact, the ones who didn't experience a renewed sense of vitality were the ones who did not follow the plan. Continue your journey and lifelong commitment to living to your fullest potential. – Debra Raybern

Congratulations! You have successfully finished your first 90 days, which included:

Month 1:
- ❑ Obtain your baseline blood work through various testing and record the results on page 22.
- ❑ You have completed the Goals Chart on page 24, so you know where you are headed.
- ❑ Successfully revamp the whole house to replace all chemically-laden products and foods with healthy alternatives.
- ❑ Chose one or a combination of eating plans to begin.

Month 2:
- ❑ Pick a cleanse and follow for at least one week.
- ❑ Continue with your new and healthy eating plan.
- ❑ Begin "My First Plan" or one of the five-day cleanses for the liver or kidney.
- ❑ Spend time thinking about and journaling your thoughts and emotions that may be hindering you from living the life you desire
- ❑ Take necessary steps to remove these hindrances.
- ❑ Add specific supplements and essential oils that support your journey to wellness.

Month 3:
- ❑ Set aside five days this month to do another five-day cleanse or other cleanse of your choice. Remember, all of the cleanses work on the whole body. The Cleansing Trio™ concentrates on the digestive system, and of course the 5-Day Liver cleanse focuses on the liver and the 5-Day Kidney on the kidneys. The others are whole body cleanses. By the end of 12 months, we hope you will have used all of the cleanses at least once. Even if this is just your second cleanse, you will have obtained great improvements by now.
- ❑ You created your own Homework for Health plan for your next 90 days.
- ❑ If you have not already, begin to Nourish with NingXia Red®, OmegaGize3™, and MultiGreens™. The supplements are taken as directed on the bottle.
- ❑ Selected and began using the essential oils.

Months 4-6: This easy to follow plan is about $200 per month and continues to help you on your journey. Be sure to keep cleansing at least five days per month for the first year. Then quarterly is generally sufficient with a healthy and nutritious diet and lifestyle. Branch out to using the many other products from Young Living.

The specific products mentioned above are for suggested starting points. As you learn your body and needs, you may need to start differently.

Maintenance Supplement ideas:

❑ NingXia Red® – one ounce per day. You may add 1-3 drops of a Vitality™ essential oil.

❑ Core Supplements™ pack – take one pack daily as suggested on the box or Master Formula™, Life 9™, Longevity™ softgels, OmegaGize³™ all taken as directed on the bottles.

❑ Essentialzyme™ or Essentialzymes-4™ or Detoxzyme® (vegan formula) taken as directed on bottle or box.

Essential Oils:

Select and use one oil from the lists on pages 68, 80 or 81 on wrists or over heart each day. Also smell the same oil twice per day for at least one minute per oil. Alternate oils so that you concentrate on a different oil each day. As you smell each oil, look at the name on the bottle and reflect on this emotion and how it may apply to you.

Emotions have profound impact on the physical body. Stress accounts for 80% of all diseases according to the American Medical Association and National Institute of Health. We must take control of all the stressors in life, both physical and emotional.

Month 4: Add the Thieves® kit of products to clean and protect you and your home from pesky germs. There are hundreds of uses for the Thieves® line to purify your home.

Month 5: Explore the skin and personal care products and select which shampoos, lotions, soaps, or more you want to try first. Keep in mind that they are highly concentrated and may last 3 months or longer. Also finish replacing the chemicals in the bathroom and throughout the home. Chemically-laden skin care products account for much of our toxic exposure. Radiant skin isn't just beautiful – its healthy – and Young Living has some of the best quality and most highly effective products.

Month 6: Purchase the Raindrop Technique® kit, Feelings™ Kit, or Golden Touch 1™ Kit. Getting one of these kits allows you to continue the essential oil learning experience. Contact an upline leader about helping you experience the Raindrop Technique®. Select and follow another cleanse. If you have not yet done the 5-Day Liver or Kidney Cleanse, one of these are good choices.

Month 7: Now that you are familiar with a sampling of the many unique and natural products from Young Living, you can start over with STEP ONE. You'll see just how far you have come and if your goals are not yet achieved, you know how to travel the wellness road.

Other must do's for the best maintenance program:

❑ Exercise at least 20 minutes per day. Be sure the type of exercise selected fits in with your ability and current state of your health. Consult a medical doctor or personal trainer if unsure.

❑ Stop using chemical cleaners, chemically-laden body care and bath products. Switch to the many products offered by Young Living. The Thieves® Household Cleaner will clean and disinfect your home safely and effectively.

❑ Stop the use of the microwave. Unplug it or, better yet, completely remove it from the kitchen. A convection toaster oven is a great alternative.

❑ Do not substitute the YL supplements or oils with those of another company. They will not give you the amazing results thousands of my (Debra) clients received.

❑ Select three supplements or oils for the top three symptoms you are experiencing. Use the *Essential Oil Desk Reference* (EODR) book to learn about the products and suggestions for your challenges. If you do not own the EODR, it is a must have for using the oils to their maximum benefit, for restoring your health, and for taking care of your family. Learn about each oil, not just the symptoms section. Explore the rest of the book as there is a wealth of knowledge to be gained.

❑ Nutrition is a must. It must be wholesome – not fast food or full of preservatives. The book *Nutrition 101: Choose Life!*, is the premier nutrition primer for all ages, and it is an excellent recipe and resource guide to help you move from unhealthy eating habits to creating a culture of healthy choices. Order online at www.growinghealthyhomes.com, Amazon, or other favorite booksellers.

❑ Begin the day with warm lemon water as a fantastic aid for digestion that supports your overall detoxification process and stimulates your digestion for the day.

Repeat again and again for a life time of wellness, energy and vitality.

Additional blank charts are available in the Resource Section or http://growinghealthyhomes.com/bookextras.

My Plan

Copy this sentence in the space below and say it out loud.
"I am well and thriving in life!"

_____

Reassess Your Physical Health:

Height:_____

Weight:_____

Body Mass Index (BMI): _____

Blood pressure: _____

Pulse: _____

Basal body temperature: _____

Reassess the Health of Your Home:

Toxins removed: _____

Healthy replacements made: _____

Other comments: _____

_____

_____

_____

Reassess the Health of Your Mind: _____

_____

_____

Reassess the Health of Your Emotions: _____

_____

_____

Month 4 plan: _____

Month 5 plan: _____

If you continue on this journey, what should you expect in:

Two weeks – Your cravings for sugar and junk foods should lessen.

60 days – All cravings eliminated, and you will feel a difference as your body fat and weight improve. Challenges that bothered you before are diminishing.

90 days – Kudos to you! The cells in your body have all turned over at least once, lots of toxins are gone, and you are well on your way to the new and improved you!

Six months – Everyone is asking you, "What are you doing? You look great!" Even if weight was not an issue, your skin will be more luminous and radiant and not just on your face. As you take control of emotions through cleansing your emotions and mind, stress will have melted away. You'll be sharing your *Road to Wellness* journey with others and may even start a *Road to Wellness* group meeting weekly or monthly to encourage others to join the healthy journey.

One year – Now you're a pro. Every organ has had its time in the spotlight and experienced at least one round of cleansing. Your home is completely free of harmful chemicals. The pantry and refrigerator have been fully made over and your repertoire of meal recipes is worthy of any wholesome cookbook.

> In my experience with thousands of clients and 12 years of consulting, the only people who did not have a good measure of success where the ones who DID NOT follow through. Your health and well-being are important for not only you, but your friends and family who all want a healthy you! – Debra Raybern

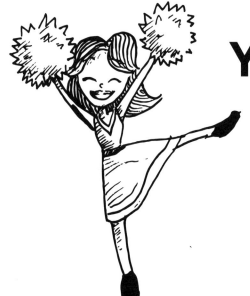

You are a winner!

> This moment – this feeling of accomplishment you've attained – it's the reason we wrote this book! We pray that you continue on this road *well*-traveled with every intention of staying the course. Look around and find those who want a better path to travel and get them started on the *Road to Wellness* too! – Laura Hopkins

Additional Considerations

Weight management

As previously discussed, a scale does not tell the extent of your health. Almost everyone will desire to lose a few pounds at some point in their life; others may find their best weight after losing 25, 50, or even 100 pounds. Following the cleansing and nourishing plan in *Road to Wellness* will help you achieve your proper weight as long as you remain committed. Starvation and fancy diet pills are short-term, dead end roads. Stick to sensible eating, cleansing, nourishing, and exercise plans for the better healthy path. Medical science has proven again and again that this path is the most effective and long lasting way to regain proper weight.

Tools to help

These products that help you burn fat and control your appetite, and you may decide to incorporate such tools to give you a jump start. Take as directed if there is no explanation listed.

- ❑ Slique™ Slim Caps
- ❑ Slique™ Protein Shake
- ❑ Slique™ Gum
- ❑ Balance Complete™
- ❑ Pure Protein Complete™
- ❑ Peppermint Vitality™ – one drop in water 30 mins before a meal; also smell before eating
- ❑ Ocotea Vitality™ – one drop in water 30 mins after a meal

Children

Our children are exposed to the same chemicals in the environment, home products and foods as we are. So, do they need a detox? Maybe so, just not to the same extent as an adult may. The best cleansing program for children includes getting the toxins out of their homes, good nutritious foods in their bodies, plenty of sleep, and appropriate exercise. The body naturally eliminates our toxic load, provided we are not putting in more in than can go out.

> It's up to parents to set the example and make the best buying choices, but children should be taught to make their own healthy choices. The reason behind their choices shouldn't be that "mom or dad told me," it should be because they want to have a healthy body. In our book, *Nutrition 101: Choose Life!* we help kids and adults understand the consequences of bad food and the benefits of good food by teaching the systems of the body and how food affects them. – Laura Hopkins

If a teenager is in overall good health, staying active and eating well, going on a three-day juice fast or a "My First Cleanse" should be just fine. In general, feed them whole foods and no junk or processed foods. Pack a healthy lunch alternative and start the school days with a healthy breakfast. Teaching kids to make healthy choices is possible. *Nutrition 101: Choose Life!* is a great way to engage all ages and help establish new healthy habits, or educate kids on how to choose the foods that their bodies need. Kids who help in the kitchen or pick out food at the grocery store or farmer's market are much more likely to experiment with new flavors, colors, and textures.

Example breakfast:

Have children help chop vegetables the day before and help store them in sealed containers. In the morning, have them pick their own vegetables to sauté in coconut oil and, if appropriate, oversee them using the stovetop. Add eggs to the pan, scramble them with the veggies, and serve it as "Confetti Eggs." Making it fun and memorable will encourage their discovery.

Example sack lunch:
Laura's daughter always enjoyed Turkey Crunchers, which was simply stick veggies like carrots, celery, or sweet peppers, wrapped in slices of turkey. She would try to guess the vegetable inside. Modify it with whatever sliced protein you like, and veggies that will have a "crunch" when you bite them. Replace prepacked chips with non-GMO popcorn or his or her favorite healthy crackers. Let the child choose from two or three fruit options to round out the meal. A vegetarian option includes a variety of crunchy vegetables and fruit dipped into protein-rich dips like hummus or almond butter.

Example dinner:
A meal like Rainbow Tacos is a family favorite. Who can add the most color in their toppings? Offer options to expose children to various colors and textures. Substitute leafy spinach or red cabbage for iceberg lettuce. Add heirloom, multi-colored tomatoes, and finely chop or shred zucchini or yellow squash for added variety. Letting kids make their own healthy choices early on gives them a better foundation for making healthy choices in the future.

Seniors
The organization known as AARP will list you as a senior starting at age 55. GASP! Most agree though that 65 is the standard threshold for that status, as it is the age when most qualify for Medicare. WHEW!

Seniors in good health and already eating a healthy whole foods diet may also cleanse. If this is your first cleanse, then as with adults of any age, start slow and work up to a full week or longer several times per year.

> Why not reach 65 in your best health ever and never NEED the Medicare you qualify for?? Novel idea? Not really. Who do you know living well into their 80's and 90's? – Debra Raybern

More and more people are living well into their mid-to-late-nineties, some even into the 100's. Debra's neighbor Miss Leona recently passed away at 95, still taking out her own trash days before. Another friend, Miss Iva, was 104 at her recent passing. Grandma Hopkins recently went to heaven at age 99, after being in good health for the majority of those years, getting physical activity daily for more than 90 years, and eating food she grew herself most of her life.

Being a senior doesn't resign you to a walker and pureed foods, NO! This is your best time. The children are grown, the nest is empty, and you have time to fulfill your later years with service to others, fun, travel, and spending time with those you love.

Begin taking care of your body now so it serves you like the ladies mentioned above, and be proud to say your age, while looking and acting 10 to 20 years younger.

Pregnancy and nursing
Pregnancy is not the time to consider a cleanse. This is the time to eat healthy as outlined in STEP THREE. Save cleansing for after the baby is born and ideally when the infant is no longer solely relying on breast milk. Once the baby is getting at least half his or her nourishment from solid or pureed foods and not just mom, then a cleanse may be considered. Select the milder My First Cleanse, or eat all raw foods and juices for a weekend to be sure it does not alter the taste of breast milk to something that a child may not like. You don't want to do anything that will stop the baby from nursing or begin to dry up the milk supply earlier than mom prefers.

If you are considering getting pregnant within the next six to 12 months, then start a cleanse now. There have been several women who struggled to get pregnant, began a cleansing routine, and were pregnant in a short time. A great resource for moms choosing to use essential oils during this time is *Gentle Babies*.

Sharing with others

You will be eager to share your successes with others! In fact, you may have people come and ask you, "What are you doing? You look so healthy?" Remember, it has taken you a year to develop a routine of cleansing and nourishing, so be mindful when you share your experiences to not suggest they just start using the Young Living oils and oil-infused products without the help of *Road to Wellness*.

Consider having new enrollees try the NingXia Red® kit before having them dive straight into the Everyday Oils collection. Wearing, smelling, or ingesting the essential oils for someone living a highly toxic life may be overwhelming and lead to a potential healing reaction they are not thrilled with such as a headache, skin rash, upset stomach or worse; in that case, you and your oils will be to blame.

Just like the authors, many of you have been enjoying Young Living products with great success and enjoyment for years. For you to routinely apply oils to the skin or ingest the Vitality™ oils orally is a breeze, but it's taken you and your body a while to detoxify. As we know, the oils themselves seek to restore and balance what is out of balance. Most people don't realize their current toxic load and what it is doing to the body. So we have a suggestion: when you enroll a new member, either gift them a copy of this book or make sure they get a copy for themselves so they can begin fully enjoying the Young Living experience.

If you start helping people use these wonderful products, you can also reap the rewards through the optional, but generous, compensation plan with Young Living. Please see our book *Road to Royal: Roadmap to Success* for details on how to maximize that journey as well.

Resources and Blank Charts

Recommended Resources

Here are our recommended resources, listed alphabetically, for your home library:

First and foremost, we recommend reading the Bible, especially for tackling buried feelings and emotional detoxing, and also to increase your faith and belief that you are fearfully and wonderfully made!

A More Excellent Way
Henry Wright – A Christian perspective on emotional healing. He does not like natural remedies, but his insight into emotional issue and physical health is excellent.

The Biology of Belief
Bruce Lipton, PhD. - Through the research of Dr. Lipton and other leading-edge scientists, stunning new discoveries have been made about the interaction between your mind and body and the processes by which cells receive information.

Chemical-Free Home I, II, and III
Melissa Poepping – Personal insights and recipes tested by multiple generations compiled into handy, compact booklets for frequent use and to give to others.

Discovery of The Ultimate Superfood
Dr. Gary Young, Ronald Lawrence MD, PhD, Marc Schreuder – Everything you ever needed to know about NingXia Red® and why it truly is the World's Most Powerful Superfood Drink.

Essential Oil Desk Reference (EODR) and Essential Oil Pocket Reference (EOPR)
Life Science Publishing – This is the reference guide to learn about the vast properties and capabilities of pure essential oils.

Essential Oils Integrative Medical Guide
D. Gary Young – Written for health professionals integrating essential oils into their practice and features many recipes Gary has used in a clinical setting.

Feelings Buried Alive Never Die
Karol K. Truman – A great quick reference tool to help match a physical symptom to an emotional pattern.

Gentle Babies: Essential Oils and Natural Remedies for Pregnancy, Childbirth and Infant Care
Debra Raybern – Be confident in knowing you can use essential oils during this special time in your life. Makes a great baby shower gift as well.

The Gift in You: Discovering New Life Through Gifts Hidden in Your Mind
Caroline Leaf, PhD. – Learn to unlock your God-given talents and eliminate the "Gift-Blockers" that hinder you from reaching your full destiny in God.

Healing Oils of the Bible
David Stewart, PhD – A detailed and fascinating compilation of Scripture and historical data about the ancient use of essential oils. This popular book comes in multiple languages and inspired a condensed booklet edition and a study format with a DVD and booklets.

Inner Transformations, Using Essential Oils
LeAnne Deardeuff, DC – Use the Young Living products to detoxify and cleanse.

Jumpstart Your Metabolism: How to Lose Weight by Changing the Way You Breathe
Pam Grout – By increasing the amount of oxygen you take in, you can help your body do a more efficient job of releasing hydrogen, the chief culprit in the storage of excess fat. You'll be amazed at the benefits of learning to breathe the right way.

Healing Oils, Healing Hands
Linda L. Smith – A retired nurse teaches about anointing with the oils for healing, as was done by the early church.

Healthy and Free: A Journey to Wellness for Your Body, Soul, and Spirit
Beni Johnson – The author received a life-changing revelation about how anyone can start walking in holistic health – including you! Jesus died for your spirit, soul, and body. This means you can experience His resurrection life in all three areas!

The Healing Power of Enzymes
DicQui Fuller Looney, PhD. – Learn how enzyme supplements can turn your life around! Lower your cholesterol, strengthen your immune system, revitalize your energy level, understand your body type, and shed excess weight.

The Law of Attraction: The Science of Attracting More of What You Want and Less of What You Don't
Michael J. Losier – With its easy-to-follow three-step formula (Identify Your Desire, Give Your Desire Attention, and Allowing), complete with tips, tools, exercises, and scripts, leaders can learn how to use the Law of Attraction deliberately and integrate it into their daily life.

Nature's Mold RX – the Non-Toxic Solution to Toxic Mold
Edward R. Close, PhD and Jacquelyn Close, RA – After having to battle mold in his own house, Dr. Close, a world recognized expert in environmental science found the Thieves® oil blend to work better and safer than any chemical. Packed full of research and a mold eradication plan.

NingXia Wolfberry: The Ultimate Superfood: How the NingXia Wolfberry and Four Other Foods Help Combat Heart Disease, Cancer, Chronic Fatigue, Depression, Diabetes and More
D. Gary Young – Discover the medicinal power of the NingXia Wolfberry and how it can constitute the key to longevity. This well-documented book uncovers the curative capabilities of the Chinese fruit to speed recovery and prolong wellness.

Nutrition 101: Choose Life!
Debra Raybern, Sera Johnson, Laura Hopkins, Karen Hopkins – Learn the 12 body systems and how food and supplements can support optimum health or not. Written for home school families but used by all families wanting to have more energy, focus, health and wellness. Suggested supplements focus on Young Living products.

Oola: Finding Balance in an Unbalanced World
Troy Amdahl and Dave Braun – Oola is not your typical self-help book. Oola is a "state of awesomeness." It's when your life is balanced and growing in the 7 key areas of life (Fitness, Finance, Family, Field, Faith, Friends, and Fun).

Releasing Emotional Patterns with Essential Oils
Carol Mein, PhD. – Excellent chart based resource to match symptoms of emotional and physical challenges with YL essential oils.

Think and Eat Yourself Smart
Caroline Leaf, PhD. – (This is the description on Amazon) Science is beginning to understand that our thinking has a deep and complicated relationship with our eating. Our thoughts before, during, and after eating profoundly impact our food choices, our digestive health, our brain health, and more. Yet most of us give very little thought to our food beyond taste and basic nutritional content.

Blank Charts

The following seven pages contain reproducible tools.

If you would like to have printer-friendly documents of many of the items listed in the Resource Section, go to http://growinghealthyhomes.com/bookextras to access the PDF downloads. You will have to create a free account with Growing Healthy Homes or log-in to an existing account to access the downloads. You have access to print these documents for your personal use through express copyright permission.

Test Results

Test	Optimal Range					
Glucose/Pancreas	70-110 mg/dl					
Fructosamine	1.20-1.60 mmol/L					
Blood urea nitrogen (BUN)	6-25 mg/dl					
Creatine	0.60-1.50 mg/dL					
Alkaline phosphatase	30-115 U/L					
Total bilirubin	0.10-1.20 mg/dl					
SGOT (AST)	0-33 U/L					
SGPT (ALT)	25					
Iron, Serum	100					
Gama Glutamyltransferase	2-65 U/L					
Total Protein	6.0-8.5 g/dl					
Total Cholesterol	180-220					
LDL	Less than 100mg/dL					
HDL	60 mg/dL and higher					
WBC White Blood Count	4,500-11,000 white blood cells per microliter (mcL)					
RBD Red Blood Count	4.5-5.1 x 106 microliter for females 4.5-5.9 x 106/ microliter for males					
TSH – Thyroid Stimulating Hormone	0.4-4.2 microunits per milliliter (mcU/mL) or 0.4-4.2 milliunits per liter (mU/L)					
T3	80-180 ng/dl					
T4	4.6-12 ug/dl					
Triglycerides	149 mg/dL or lower					

Medications

Medicine	Why	Body System(s)	Date Began	Date Ended

Health Goals

Challenge	Body System Affected	How long/Priority	Solutions

Room-by-Room Toxin Removal

ROOM:		
	Product(s) found	**Replaced with**
Ammonia		
Chlorine		
Fluoride		
Glycol ethers		
PERC		
PFCs		
Phthalates		
Propylene glycol		
Quats		
NaOH		
Sulfates		
Triclosan		

ROOM:		
	Product(s) found	**Replaced with**
Ammonia		
Chlorine		
Fluoride		
Glycol ethers		
PERC		
PFCs		
Phthalates		
Propylene glycol		
Quats		
NaOH		
Sulfates		
Triclosan		

Unhealthy Food Replacement

Meal	Ingredients to Replace	Healthier Options

Track Your Nutrients

		Monday	Tuesday	Wednesday	Thursday	Friday	Saturday	Sunday	Totals
Protein	Breakfast								
	Lunch								
	Dinner								
Fiber	Breakfast								
	Lunch								
	Dinner								
Sugar	Breakfast								
	Lunch								
	Dinner								
Fat	Breakfast								
	Lunch								
	Dinner								

		Monday	Tuesday	Wednesday	Thursday	Friday	Saturday	Sunday	Totals
Protein	Breakfast								
	Lunch								
	Dinner								
Fiber	Breakfast								
	Lunch								
	Dinner								
Sugar	Breakfast								
	Lunch								
	Dinner								
Fat	Breakfast								
	Lunch								
	Dinner								

Oils for Emotions

Oil	Emotion	Worn/Diffused	Words of Affirmation

About the Authors

Road to Wellness packs much of Debra's clinical experience and Laura's practical insights into a guide every family can take to truly live the abundantly healthy and vibrant life they desire.

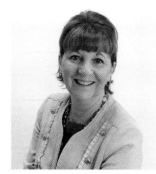

Debra Raybern

www.debraraybern.com

Christian Naturopath, Master Herbalist, Certified Nutritional Counselor, Internationally Certified Aroma Therapist, Author, Speaker, and Young Living Royal Crown Diamond.

Debra has been sharing natural health care solutions using traditional naturopathic and herbal remedies in conjunction with proper, body system specific nutrition since 1992. She has been a contributing writer for several publications such as *Countryside, Home School Digest, This Old Schoolhouse, The Link,* and *An Encouraging Word*. Debra is a popular speaker at expos, trade shows, church and civic groups, midwifery and homeschool conferences speaking on herbal first aid, God's herbs and essential oils as natural alternatives, nutrition, family health, and more.

Her book *Gentle Babies* is helping woman enjoy the special time of pregnancy, childbirth and caring for newborns. *Nutrition 101: Choose Life!* co-authored with Sera Johnson, Laura Hopkins, and Karen Hopkins, is fast becoming the most sought after "nutrition" program for families to teach sound nutritional practices at an early age. Debra's book *Road to Royal* is a business builders dream book with proven strategies to help anyone achieve success sharing a healthy lifestyle with the Young Living products.

Though she has retired from private consulting, Debra continues to share her passion for health and wellness in God's healing and restoring power of natural herbs, essential oils and nutrition through seminars, books, and articles. Her vast knowledge, experience, and Godly anointing allows her the privilege to help countless people with both minor and life threatening health problems by educating them in healthy nutrition practices and lifestyles to cleanse and promote the body to heal itself.

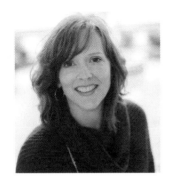

Laura Hopkins
Thrivensity.com

As a wife, homeschooling mother, author, active volunteer, and professional communicator with nearly two decades of experience in the public and private sectors, Laura loves combining her passion for her family with her gifts and talents in writing and education.

She and her husband, Jonathan, are Young Living Diamonds and the cofounders of Thrivensity, Inc., through which they encourage thousands of people around the world to thrive intensely in mind, body, and spirit. When she is not speaking at a seminar, leading a small group of children at church, or anything in between, sharing the love of God by feeding His beloved and teaching them about His food remains one of her favorite pastimes.

To further assist others on their wellness journeys, Laura co-authored *Nutrition 101: Choose Life!* and *Road to Wellness*, collaborated with Debra Raybern on *Road to Royal*, and edited four additional books published by Growing Healthy Homes LLC. She also has written for the Oral Roberts University Alumni magazine.

Her favorite essential oil blend is Transformation™ because "it smells phenomenal" and also embodies Romans 12:2: "Do not be conformed to this world, but be transformed by the renewing of your mind that you may prove that good, acceptable, and perfect will of God."

To obtain additional copies of *Road to Wellness* and for more information on other books by Growing Healthy Homes, please visit our website at www.GrowingHealthyHomes.com

Nutrition 101: Choose Life!

Gentle Babies

Gentle Babies Quick Reference Handout Pack

Gentle Babies DVD

The ABC's of Building a Young Living Organization

Young Living Skincare Product Handout Pack

Notes

Notes

Notes